BEYOND THE RED ZONE

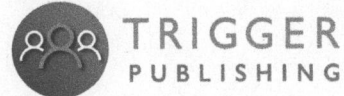

BEYOND THE RED ZONE

"I've always said how important it is to protect your mentals." **Marshawn Lynch, former NFL running back and Super Bowl XLVIII champion**

"BJ's lived experience is a shining example to society and the next generation to never give up on your dreams. BJ shows us all that by 'Leaving No One Behind', there is always hope and light despite the times of darkness. BJ's story unlocks a treasure trove of wisdom from those who've walked the same path. Brace yourself for a confidence-boosting, hope-infused journey that inspires and showcases the importance of mental health wellbeing and prosperity." **Kyle Walker, captain of Manchester City Football Club and member of the England national football team**

"BJ proves that stepping up, opening up and leading by example can change and create a world that Leaves No One Behind." **Marquel Blackwell, running backs coach at Texas A&M**

"A game-changer for mental health, BJ goes far beyond advocacy. A leading voice and icon for the next generation." **Yusuf Shakir, football operations assistant at the University of Florida and former head football coach at Lincoln High School**

ABOUT THE AUTHOR

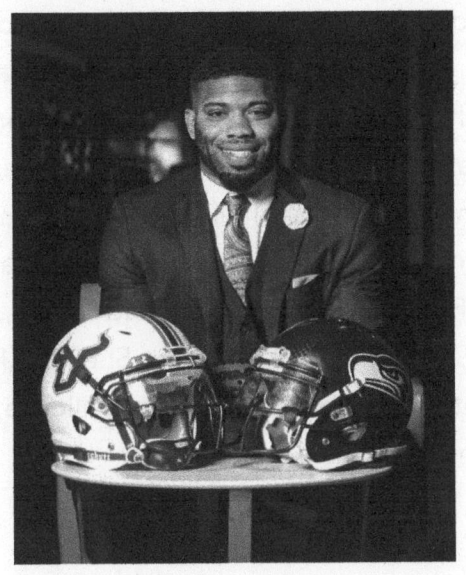

BJ Daniels is a former professional football player and passionate mental health advocate. His career began at the University of South Florida, where he started as quarterback for all four years and still holds a record as the Big East's second all-time yardage leader. In the 2013 NFL draft, BJ was selected in the seventh round by the San Francisco 49ers. Shortly thereafter, he was waived by the 49ers and picked up by the Seattle Seahawks, with whom he won Super Bowl XLVIII over the Denver Broncos. He also played for the Houston Texans, New York Giants, Chicago Bears and Atlanta Falcons.

Now, BJ has returned to his roots and works at USF as the Assistant Director of Donor, Community and Alumni Engagement in Development, and is also the head of the USF Athletics Alumni Association. He has made it his mission to use his lived experience in football – both the positive lessons and difficult realities of life on the gridiron – to inspire international change in the way we talk about and deal with mental health. He is the Global Ambassador for TriggerHub, which has taken his trademarked mantra, "Leave No One Behind", from Florida to Sheffield, UK, where it is emblazoned across the jerseys of four professional sports teams: Sheffield Wednesday Football Club, the Sheffield Sharks, the Sheffield Steelers and, starting in fall 2024, the Sheffield Hatters. He is also a sought-after public speaker on resilience, adaptability and mental health.

BEYOND THE RED ZONE

HOW A SUPER BOWL WINNER BECAME A MENTAL HEALTH CHAMPION

BJ DANIELS

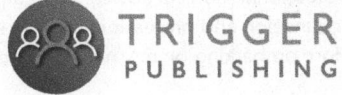

Published in 2024 by Trigger Publishing
An imprint of Shaw Callaghan Ltd

UK Office
The Stanley Building
7 Pancras Square
Kings Cross
London N1C 4AG

US Office
On Point Executive Center, Inc
3030 N Rocky Point Drive W
Suite 150
Tampa, FL 33607
www.triggerpublishing.com

Text Copyright © 2024 BJ Daniels
Design and layout © 2024 Shaw Callaghan Ltd

BJ Daniels has asserted his moral right to be identified as the author of this Work in accordance with the Copyright Designs and Patents Act 1988.

All rights reserved. No part of this publication may be reproduced, stored in a retrieval system, or transmitted in any form or by any means, electronically, mechanical, photocopying, recording or otherwise, without the prior permission of the copyright owners and the publishers.

A CIP catalogue record for this book is available upon
request from the British Library
ISBN: 978-1-83796-477-2
Ebook ISBN: 978-1-83796-092-7

Trigger Publishing encourages diversity and different viewpoints. However, all views, thoughts and opinions expressed in this book are the author's own and are not necessarily representative of us as an organization.

All material in this book is set out in good faith for general guidance and no liability can be accepted for loss or expense incurred in following the information given. In particular this book is not intended to replace expert medical or psychiatric advice. It is intended for informational purposes only and for your own personal use and guidance. It is not intended to act as a substitute for professional medical advice. The author is not a medical practitioner nor a counselor, and professional advice should be sought if desired before embarking on any health-related program.

For my family.

For my family

CONTENTS

Introduction   xiii

1   Super Bowl Champion BJ Daniels   1
2   My Fire Truck   19
3   I'm Short, I'm Black, I'm a Quarterback   31
4   The Other Side of the Tracks   41
5   Seventh Round   61
6   A Dream Come True… Kind of   77
7   Keeping Up with the Joneses   93
8   "You Played Well Today, Son"   115
9   Sleepless in Seattle   135
10   The Struggle to Survive   157
11   A Dream Realized   181
12   My Faith   203
13   Leave No One Behind   213

Acknowledgments   229
References   231

INTRODUCTION

I've been in what feels like a thousand hotel rooms. As I stand by its window, this room is as familiar as that feeling raging deep inside me. My bag is packed on the bed. It almost packs itself now. Training gear folded, cleats laced; both sit on another overnight change of clothes. The neutral colors of the room's walls and bedding are designed to be subtle, but that's not me, not today. Today is about showing my colors, my drive, the fire that sees me continue to pursue a dream. Today is another day of NFL tryouts. Another training camp in another city with another team in our National Football League. Today is another trial, me asking a coach to see something, to acknowledge what I might offer. Today, once again, I chase my goal and show the fire inside me. Soon, I'll arrive, that jersey will go on, and all eyes will be on me. Can I be the player they want? *Let me show you.*

***

Growing up, all I wanted was to be a quarterback in the NFL. I had fallen in love with football, and from a young age, watching the college game with my dad in my hometown of Tallahassee, I had been mesmerized by these godlike sportsmen, men who I couldn't wait to one day emulate when I made the step up as a pro.

It started with life's first steps. A ball was placed in my hands – a basketball first. The simple fun that could be found in its bounce. Then, the thrill of dunking on a small hoop in our living room. Both my father and his brother played college basketball, and it was that game that started my love affair with sports. But then came football: the hits, the speed, the sheer vastness of the space, and what could be achieved with a combination of strength, pace and intelligence.

It was in elementary school that I began to play the game seriously. There, I first put on my armor – the pads, the helmet. Suddenly, I was the same as the men I had watched play on the college campus where my family lived when I was born. With that armor on, running onto the field, I quickly realized, with the ball in my hands, that this was my place.

I wasn't there for the big hits, and I wasn't there to run. Don't get me wrong, I was fine with the physicality of the game, and I was always a good athlete who could run with the best of them. But it was holding the ball, seeing what was in front of me, and sending that ball forward that appealed to me from a very young age.

"I'm a quarterback." They were words that rolled off my tongue with pride and ease. I reveled in the position, the responsibility, the notion that it is on you to move your team forward. You bring to life the coaches' wishes, you are the catalyst for progress, and to be at the heart of the

INTRODUCTION

offensive game, having to call the play and create havoc in your opponent's defense, was something that appealed to my competitive and aggressive (in a sporting sense) nature.

Because of my passion to play in that position, life lessons came at me quicker and harder than any defensive linesman; the decision-makers, be they in grade school, college or the NFL, were there to sack me, too. But, like any quarterback worthy of the position, I had to keep getting up. There is always another play, and you have to keep the game – and your dreams – moving forward.

Sports teach you to take life's setbacks. Within a game, the hits come fast, momentum and yardage are lost, defense and offense must work together if points are to be scored. From a young age, my struggle to persuade coaches to play me in the position I so adamantly felt was my best was a never-ending battle to gain their trust.

Making your dreams come true is never simple. The struggle to get to the top of the mountain must be part of the fun. It must be every bit as pleasing and rewarding as the supposedly clean air at the summit. I say "supposedly" because reaching that summit and living your dream isn't always what you envision, and in this book, I want to tell my story, one which saw me work and struggle to make my dream come true, only to realize that the work and struggle never end.

Today, I own a Super Bowl ring. I was involved in three Super Bowls, and the trinket given to me in 2014, when my team, the Seattle Seahawks, beat the Denver Broncos, brings me great pleasure. It was won alongside great men, making up a great team, and I will never forget any of them, but as my story will show, I now look back on the work I did to keep my place in a notoriously ruthless NFL, and take equal or even greater pride in it.

Life as a pro athlete is both short and multilayered. The fans and the public only get to see the games. The games are, of course, the pinnacle of the working week, everything that us athletes strive for and will be judged on. That's only right, but what people don't see, and what I hope this book will shed light on, is both the work that went into getting the opportunity to play, the insecurities that go with trying to keep that opportunity, and the dark places that athletes can go when the floodlights are turned off.

Glory, adoration, fame and fortune – these are the presumed side effects of signing a first contract in the NFL. Anyone who tells you that they are not a welcome part of making it as pro is lying, and while the very thought of them can spin a young man's head – this now slightly older man will testify to that – the sport will spit you out should they become your sole reason for being there.

All I wanted to do, from a young age, was play. Put those pads on, put a helmet on, and go out there and play. But even as that Super Bowl ring slid onto my finger, I couldn't say my goal was achieved. It was an incredible thrill – in my rookie year – to be so involved with what is the pinnacle of the game, but it didn't change my almost childlike desire to simply play.

In these pages I will tell my story, of the desire that saw me move from city to city, staying in hotel after hotel, living

INTRODUCTION

out of a small suitcase, trying to show people my worth, and how that yearning to play the game spurred me on, driving me over miles and miles, from Seattle to New York and everywhere in between.

On each occasion, with each team, in front of each coach judging me, the easy part was having the ball in my hand. Throwing, running, playing – that would never ever grow tiring. However, the constant eyes on us players giving our all to make teams, please people and change our own beliefs, the heavy expectations put upon us, and the stereotypes that influenced the decisions made – that began to wear thin. Facing defensive lines and throwing touchdowns was the goal, but keeping my focus, regardless of the obstacles placed in front of me, that was the key, and trust me, it wasn't easy.

Today, I look back on my career and the work ethic that took me to the highest echelons of football with immense pride. There are no regrets. From a young age, I worked as hard as I could, I was courteous and polite to even those who tried to hinder my efforts, but – and this is the key – I stayed true to myself.

Now, with my faith, and through my work teaching and talking to young people, I can look back and acknowledge my time in the world of elite sports, take what I learned and tie it to their everyday lives. Whatever their goals, I emphasize that by staying true to themselves, working hard and refusing to bow to what others presume is best for them, they can be the best version of themselves and change the world.

I look back at that young man, standing in yet another hotel room, his bag packed but his dreams still raging. I want to tell him to keep going, I want to tell him that it's all worth it, I want to tell him I'm proud. My story isn't all about the glory of sports, but how my desire to make an impact molded and shaped me. *Let me show you.*

1

SUPER BOWL CHAMPION BJ DANIELS

THE TRUTH BEHIND THE RING

Hello, I'm Super Bowl winner BJ Daniels. Don't worry, I wouldn't always introduce myself this way, but since winning one of those famous rings our National Football League gives out to their ultimate champions, I have noticed that it's the first thing new people want to talk about.

I don't blame them. I have always loved sports, have always wanted to excel at whatever game I played. And the game I played most was football. To me, from a young age, the football field was a place I could cherish, a place that my deep competitiveness found its home, a place where I could fully be myself.

I grew up studying great athletes, watching how they were on the field, what made them tick, considering what made them great. Because of college football players such as Charlie Ward, a man I watched and cheered on as a kid with my dad at Florida State University, and Virginia Tech quarterback Michael Vick, who I admired so much that I wore his number, 7, on my jersey, I have been interested in what makes these people propel themselves from mortal men to superheroes.

When people meet me and immediately want to know about winning the Super Bowl, I get it. I get the intrigue. I get that they want to know more about how it feels to be part of the team that climbs the ultimate mountain, how a winner celebrates the achievement and, of course, where I keep the ring.

So, let's get it out of the way: Super Bowl XLVIII, 2014.

It was getting late when we, the winners, arrived at the most exclusive club in the most exclusive city in the world. We'd done our post-game duties, we'd given the press our words of joy, we'd looked into a million television cameras and showed the world our beaming smiles. The locker room had been cleared, and soon there would be no trace of the raucous celebrations that had covered the walls and floors with both our post-game sweat and fizzy champagne. All that was left to do was party.

We arrived at New York City's most exclusive club, 1 OAK, as the Seattle Seahawks, champions of the world. We had partied before – of course we had. On countless occasions, we would go out as a team, in whatever town we might have been in, and find the best place to party. But on this night, we were a team who had reached the ultimate goal in football, so this party was just for us.

The red carpet, lined by velvet VIP ropes, awaited us. We arrived, dressed in our best, and walked along the carpet, photographers' cameras lighting our way. Then, we saw them: A-listers lining the carpet, stars from music, movies and television, and they were there to celebrate with us. The bouncers paused the line of celebrities to let the Super Bowl winners in first, so some of the most famous faces on the planet, the likes of Meek Mill and Teyana Taylor, were there as I walked by. Inside, the club was packed, but I somehow managed to spot Drake – who invited me to party at his table. (I had met Drake before at a Seahawks practice and started a conversation with him because we have the same birthday. He remembered me, and that's why he called me over that night.)

So, check this out: I was just a rookie who, in his first turbulent months in the league of my dreams, had already been on two huge teams – the Seahawks and the San Francisco 49ers – and seen very quickly how hard life could be as a pro. And then there I was, wearing that new ring, holding a glass of champagne and talking to Drake, who wanted to know how it felt to be the best.

It felt good, but it wasn't the reason I had always dreamed of going pro. There had been no childhood dreams about winning the Super Bowl, no yearning to experience the glory of the game's ultimate prize.

No, all my dreams were simply about becoming an NFL player, making it into the pro game. From elementary and middle school, into varsity football and college, I was a young quarterback who, while too often being told all the reasons why I didn't fit the role, refused to listen. Tell me why I can't do something, and I am simply going to work harder, be stronger, throw further. With that resolution I allowed myself to dream of defying the doubters. And so, when I dreamed, my mind didn't go to specific games, not to the Super Bowl, but to throwing that crucial pass or rushing those final yards as a pro quarterback.

But there I was, with the eyes of New York on me and the rest of the Seahawks, glamour all around us, and like so many of my teammates, I was a long way from home. The great thing about that squad was that so many of us had made our way to victory through many trials and tribulations. We all understood each other's battles, what it took to get to the very top.

My journey had started on the campus of Florida State University, in the state's capital, Tallahassee. My father worked there, and while I always thought I would play college football there, they – like coaches as far back as middle school – thought I was wrong. I had excelled at many other sports, especially basketball. You could really put me in any sport, and I would strive to be the best, but it was playing quarterback on a football field that felt the most like home. That position was where I knew I belonged, and no amount of doubting voices could put out the fire burning inside me to be a success at it.

More on that later, but for now, that drive had gotten me and my teammates to the Super Bowl in New York City. The choice of venue that year seemed more than perfect to me, a rookie who was suddenly experiencing an event like no other on Earth.

Strangely, New York had actually beaten Tampa that year for the right to host the league's finale. It had crossed my mind that playing a Super Bowl in the city of Tampa, a place so familiar to me, a stadium in which I had seen so many games, and a place so near my home, would have been perfect. But then when you experience just how big the Super Bowl is, and all the glitz that goes with the occasion, it was clear that New York City was perfect.

I have always considered myself a big-city type of guy. It isn't something I can say is genetic in me. My mother, for example, is from a small town in Alabama. She loves the outdoors and tending to a garden in the backyard, but I never had those interests. Give me bright lights and the big city anytime.

When I was in middle school in Tallahassee, there was a school trip planned to New York. I was so excited. This was my chance to visit the city I had only seen in films, books and on TV, and heard about in songs by my favorite musicians. But my parents said no – it was too expensive. Being young, I didn't care about all that. I was going to miss out, and I was hot.

A few years earlier, I had been in elementary school when the images of 9/11 shocked our country and the whole world. The size of the buildings coming down didn't seem real to me. I had been to cities in Florida, but I had never seen towers so high, and to see them fall, in my young eyes, didn't seem possible.

It seemed to me that there was no place like New York, no city on the planet like it, and then there I was, traveling there for a shot at the Super Bowl. I hadn't made that middle school trip, but now I was on my way with other dreams on my mind.

We arrived in New York on the Sunday prior to the game against the Denver Broncos. Being based in Washington State, the Seahawks would always make early travel arrangements to deal with the inevitable jetlag, and for a Super Bowl on the other side of the country, a week's preparation seemed reasonable.

Elite sport is all about routine. Meetings, recovery, more meetings, practice, meetings, more practice and some more recovery. Then repeat. For the biggest game of your life, a team will try to keep to some sort of normality, but truth be told, and as great as our head coach, Pete Carroll, and his staff were, you could not disguise the fact or the feeling that this was all so different.

As soon as you land in the city hosting the Super Bowl, you sense that it's showtime. It's like eating spaghetti all season and then suddenly being served lobster. But the hard thing is you have to suppress your taste buds, remain calm, stay focused and keep your mind on the game, but to be honest, that's easier said than done. The world is hovering over you, and that world is completely crazy.

You have to remember that I was new to the NFL, a rookie getting used to living his dream, whose life had moved at breakneck speed over a matter of six months. I always backed my ability, always, and I always understood the work that had to go in to move that ability along. But to have gone from wondering if I'd even make the NFL draft just months before to being part of *the* biggest sporting event in the world – well, I'm only human, and this was wild.

Pete Carroll knew it too. He had assembled a fine team, a group of men who looked out for each other and held one another accountable for everything we did. The great thing about Pete is how relaxed he is. He is a fun-loving man, and that wasn't going to change, even in the biggest week of his career.

He was so honest with us, building up a level of trust between coach and player that made everything else tick, and because of that, it was so easy to quickly fall under his wing. That's what I did. Without question. During the regular season, our work didn't feel like work. Pete made everything so fun, so no one wanted to slack because that meant missing out.

It was the same in New York. Yes, there was so much more to do – the NFL functions, the media requirements, and everything in between – but Pete helped us stay focused by keeping it normal, and that meant keeping us all smiling and relaxed.

We had everything buzzing around us, but there were still those meetings, still the playbook to learn, still the practice sessions to excel in. The thing is, with a crazy week like that, as an athlete, you have to ask yourself some questions: *Why am I here? Is it to enjoy the experience, or is it to win the damn game?*

Pete and his staff drummed it into us: *Focus on one week, and we can be set up for the rest of our lives.* With that motto firmly on our minds, the craziest of weeks slowly became more zen. We couldn't have been more together as a group. We had an attitude that was both enjoyable but, to paraphrase that great New Yorker Chuck D, one that refused to let anyone believe the hype.

We had to think that our team was bigger than that hype. Yes, we could make this the most memorable week, but not for the sake of showmanship – for each other and the goals we had worked so hard for. We had to be present, be teammates, and we believed the rewards would come.

It was all about the guys we were sitting there with, who all wanted the same thing and were there for the same reason. I have been on teams where individuals were there for different reasons. The fame, the money, the girls, the glory... everyone after different things, and it showed on the field. With Pete Carroll's Seahawks, of course there might have been a fondness for those perks, but the team was about not letting anyone down. If someone went out and partied too hard and wasn't ready to practice the next morning, then the disappointment from his teammates was far worse and far more likely to focus the mind than anything a screaming coach could dish out.

Being the back-up quarterback, I was on a team within a team, and that ethic of togetherness was even more vital and strong within our group. The three of us – Tarvaris Jackson, Russell Wilson and myself – were all so different in terms of our ages, stages in our lives and careers, and personalities, but we all supported one another, and like the rest of the team, we held each other accountable.

For all of us, it was our first time at the Super Bowl. We could relate to each other about how consuming it could be if we let it. We understood how the others were feeling; we understood the paths we had taken, the work we put as kids, teenagers and in college; and how all of it had brought us to this moment. The hurt, the rejection, the scholarships, getting cut, getting drafted (eventually), the family and friend dynamics that were affected by our careers, and now, here we all were. We all understood that the pressures that came with getting to where we wanted to be, and we strived to help each other enjoy where our hard work had gotten us.

Russell, the starting quarterback, was a fine athlete. He had played pro baseball in Colorado before breaking into the NFL with the Seahawks in 2012. Russell was his own man, but like me, he is 5-foot-11, and like me, he had experienced doubts about his height and stature for the position. But by throwing 26 touchdowns in his first season, he tied Peyton Manning's record for the most thrown by a rookie. His progress and form only proved that you didn't have to fit the mold to play quarterback at the very top level.

One thing that Russell had to deal with more than us in the regular season, as our starting quarterback, was the media attention. During Super Bowl week, though, with the world's press converging on New York, that intensity was something we all dealt with. I was used to talking to journalists, I was used to television cameras – that's part of college sports, too – but Super Bowl week is just bigger, more in your face, and you had to stay focused.

Suddenly, on media days, there was a room of new faces, reporters we'd never seen at a regular-season game – not the people we had grown to trust. We quickly learned that they were trying to set us up. If this was the biggest sporting spectacle in the world, then the press sent to cover it were going to try to find the biggest, juiciest story. It became clear they wanted something from us, something negative about a teammate – how I thought I should be starting, or maybe some trash-talk about one of our opponents. I might have been a rookie, but I wasn't born yesterday, so I side-stepped anything inappropriate.

I certainly didn't resent their attention or their methods. I understood it. I understood the magnitude of the occasion and how the world worked. I had loved football since as far back as I could remember, and while my true passion came with what I could do with the ball in my hand, watching the big games had always been part of it, too.

Actually, that's not true. Not always. Growing up with my parents in Florida, Sundays were always about church and family. My mom wouldn't have it any other way. My sisters certainly weren't interested in football like I was, and my mom would insist on a big family dinner. We would go to church, and then it was all about the food on our table and us enjoying time together.

My dad would put the games on, but it was very much background noise. He would be focused on cleaning the house, readying it and us for the coming week, and while I would keep an eye on what was happening, there was always homework that still needed to be done, and I wasn't going to be allowed to sit and lazily watch.

That was okay. Even as a kid, I was much more interested in college games and not so much an NFL fan. I mean, I liked it, but I felt that it lacked the passion of college football, which, to me, was better to watch, more dynamic, more likely to entertain.

As I got older, I did begin to take more and more of an interest in NFL games. In my teens, I would study the great quarterbacks and look at how they carried themselves. And while I was in Tampa playing quarterback at the University of South Florida, I saw first-hand how excited a city gets when the Super Bowl rolls into town.

In 2009, the Pittsburgh Steelers faced the Arizona Cardinals in Tampa, and it was such a thrill to see all the fans, from all over the country, in so many different teams' jerseys. It quickly dawned on me that this might be a game between two teams facing off to win the year's ultimate prize, but it was also a celebration of the sport, and the whole country – and world – was invited.

As I mentioned earlier, when I was young, and certainly when I was at USF witnessing the Super Bowl coming to Tampa, I still didn't dream that one day, I would be part of it. Sure, I might have played *Madden* and created myself as a player throwing the championship-winning touchdown back, but my ambition was never to be in the big game. I just wanted to play the game, be successful and make it as a pro.

One thing those video-game Super Bowls didn't deal with was trying to sleep the night before the game. All week, having arrived in New York the Sunday before, I had rested well. There was so much to do every day, and I was sleeping a good eight hours each night. Monday, Tuesday, Wednesday, all fine, but then we got closer, and suddenly it was Saturday night, and it hit me a little different: *There are no more days. The game is tomorrow.*

I spent Saturday night picking my outfit, and I wasn't the only one. We knew we were going to get photographed before and after the game, and being young, I wanted to get this right. Photographs last forever, and I didn't want to be sitting with my grandkids on my knee one day, showing them snapshots of my career, and come across a photo that made us all cringe.

Because this was my first Super Bowl, I went all out. The right jacket, the right shirt, the right tie to complement them both. I have to admit that I made it to two more Super Bowls, and on each occasion, my outfits became less formal and more casual. Maybe you get cooler as you get older.

But then it was time to turn off the lights, and I can't imagine that many of the players fell straight to sleep. The game ran through my mind, the things that might happen, the things I hoped would happen, and of course the things that I hoped would not. As the back-up quarterback, I naturally thought of Russell Wilson getting injured early in the game, forcing me to go on. I wouldn't ever wish that on a teammate, and I certainly didn't hope he'd play badly or get hurt, but I had to be focused on the fact that, at any time, I could be called up. My mind needed to be just as ready as my body.

With what felt like very little sleep, I was concerned with how I'd feel that morning, but as I got up, met with teammates, and later headed to the stadium, the adrenaline kicked in, and I felt like I could run through a brick wall. Seeing the then MetLife Stadium loom over the horizon, our NYPD police escort flanking our bus, I thought to myself, *You are here. This is it.*

A wild pop-up city of media tents, every food stand known to mankind, fan zones, kids' events, people from all over the country wearing their team jerseys – it was so much more than a game of football. I was about to take part in a global event, a phenomenon that seemed a universe away from those Friday-night high school games and weekend college matchups that I loved. All the work I put in on those nights, the competitive drive that made me excel in those arenas, we had all been through that, and that work and the love for what we did had brought us here.

I thought of my family. My girlfriend had traveled to New York to be with me, but my parents were unable to make the trip. That was hard, but we had FaceTimed nearly every day, and I knew they were with me – not physically, but my pathway to this moment had been very much theirs too. My father, on the Saturday night before the game, had seen a calm in my expression. It was one he'd seen before, one that told him I was okay – no need to worry about BJ.

In the locker room before the game, as they had throughout the week, the staff tried to bring some form of normality. We had traveled to play the Giants during the regular season, so we knew our surroundings a little, but otherwise, it was just about going through our usual routines, trying to take the same routes prior to getting out on the field.

Players were getting taped up, going through their stretches, praying, listening to music, and that all felt familiar. But deep down, we all knew that things were very different. We were all having our own internal conversations, and that was okay. But soon we would huddle up, the coaches would go through their instructions and motivational words, and then we were no longer individuals but a team, a group of players made one by a shared goal.

A lot of people might wonder how I, as a back-up quarterback, motivated myself and stayed focused while watching the biggest game of my life from the sidelines. First of all, of course everyone wants to play. That competitive spark that had lit up when I was a little boy had spread like a forest fire, so the desire to be out on the field with my teammates raged.

But here's the thing: That night, like any other as the back-up quarterback, I had to keep my positive energy. I fully understood my role within that team, and not only did I have to be ready and prepared to go on at any given time, but I had to be analyzing the game. I had to be mindful of the rhythm of the game, and every time Russell came off the field, I could offer advice, let him know how I thought the defense was trying to stop us.

That's not always the way, though. A lot of players, in my opinion, go into games with jealousy, and that jealousy brings distractions. If you don't fully know or appreciate your role, and therefore stop helping the team or a teammate, you will become negative, and you can start to wish for bad things to happen. Instead, you have to show a certain level of maturity, so that, if the moment comes when you are on that field, you will be ready to perform – you will be ready to go.

When the game started, it was clear that only one team was ready to go, and it was the Seahawks. Twelve seconds into the game, on Denver's first offensive play, their center snapped the ball back past the great Peyton Manning and into the end zone, resulting in a quick 2–0 lead. As *The New York Times* put it, "It began with a safety on the Broncos' first offensive play, which, as omens go, was akin to a black cat opening an umbrella beneath a ladder in Denver's locker room."

The start set the tone for the game, and we went into halftime with a 22-point lead. So much had been made of the Broncos as an attacking force. This was the highest-scoring team in NFL history, with a sheer offensive power capable of blowing away any team. The Seahawks weren't just "any team", though. If you told our defense they'd be blown away – a defense that, like our whole team, wanted nothing but to prove doubters wrong – you were going to get a force. That was what the Broncos came across that night in New York: a force.

Denver didn't get anything on the scoreboard until 45 minutes into the game, and the eventual 43–8 final score was the third-greatest margin of victory in Super Bowl history. It's strange when you are winning a game easily, when you know way before the last play that your team is going to win. There might be the temptation to give high fives, to be playing the big man, but you have to show respect.

I knew some of the Denver team. I had played college football and graduated with the Denver cornerback, Kayvon Webster. I cared about him, and I certainly was and am not one to gloat. Also, we're talking about Peyton Manning, a Hall of Famer, a player I had grown up watching and admiring. Being cocky in front of Peyton Manning? Not a chance.

So, there I was, standing in a New York club with Drake asking me how it felt to be a Super Bowl winner. I can't recall what I told him. The night is a bit of a blur. What I can tell you is I certainly couldn't have told him anything concrete. There had been no time to digest what we had achieved, and the truth is, ten years later, I am still unpacking it.

It seems like a long time ago, and I have the ring, a piece of jewelry to show future generations, but I don't *have* it. My mom holds onto it. I almost lost it once. I was in a crowd of people, and I was showing off. People wanted to see it, take a picture with it, so I took it off my finger to show to a young lady. I handed it to her, turned my back for a second, and the next thing I knew, she was gone.

Luckily for me, one of my closest friends was standing at the door. He saw the whole thing, took the ring back from the girl and returned it to me. As for the girl, she disappeared into the crowd. At the time, I was in a panic, but now I wonder if the ring itself is important.

Don't get me wrong, I'll always cherish it. But I cherish the memories of being there, I cherish my teammates, what we achieved together and how we proved our worth far more. The ring we all have may sparkle, but nothing will ever shine as bright as the effort that went into getting there and winning it.

Leading up to the game, all week, the team had been told to focus. "Focus and you'll be set up for life." So, am I set up for life? That question I still can't answer, but what I do know is there is so much more to my life in football than touchdowns and Super Bowl rings. Making it in elite pro sport is hard. The pressures and the disappointments are all part of being in it, but I have seen the dark places where some people end up. I've seen the darkness that some men couldn't find their way back from.

So, nice to meet you. Yes, I am NFL Super Bowl winner BJ Daniels, but this story is about so much more...

2

MY FIRE TRUCK

A DETERMINED MIND WILL ALWAYS FIGURE IT OUT

2

When I was a young boy, four or five maybe, my favorite toy was a fire truck. Red and shiny, I loved that truck. I'd roll it along my apartment's floor, up and down, putting out imaginary fires and helping my imaginary community for hours and hours. My real community, due to my dad's work as a resident attendant, was the Florida State University campus, and our neighbors were students. It wasn't long before I noticed them, what they were doing, how they acted, and one thing caught my eye. Maybe I was getting too old for that fire truck.

One day, I went to my parents and asked for a skateboard. I saw this mode of transport on campus, watched with awe as the students whizzed around, getting to and from class, with the odd trick thrown in for good measure. Yes, that was the new toy I wanted. It was time for that fire truck and its imaginary precinct to go out of service. So, I went to my mom and dad.

"No chance, you're too young." There was no discussion, no negotiation, just a mutual decision that their little boy was too little, too young to be trusted with his first set of wheels. Devastated, I walked away from them and into my room, only to watch from the window as the students passed by, the sound of their spinning skateboard wheels taunting me. I wanted one so bad. *No chance, you're too young.* The words hung in my little room, and then I looked in the corner, and there it was: my fire truck. An idea formed in my mind.

Outside of our apartment, there was a hill. To me, it seemed mountainous, but looking back, it was a small, fairly steep hill on which the students strolled up and down on their way to class. I would play there too, and that day, I took my fire truck and headed to the hill's peak. The truck was big enough to stand on and, I hoped, take my weight. So, I stepped on top, and with a gentle push, I was off.

For what seemed like hours that day, I was up and down, the wheels on the firetruck wearing thin from their newfound duties. In my mind, the college students stood and marveled at my invention, maybe even the ones on skateboards. Up and down I went, and I came back again and again for days. But then I got braver.

Could I go faster? Could I look even cooler to those students? Previously, I had just used one push to head down the hill. But why not, while heading down, give it another push? Not a good idea. With no brakes on the truck, I went too fast, lost control, flew off and scraped myself pretty bad – at least, I thought it was pretty bad at the time. My mom cleaned me up, and while they weren't going to show too much sympathy for my overzealousness, both she and my dad saw and admired my determination, and soon after that, I got a skateboard.

I'm not sure where that determination came from, but it has been there my whole life. It's a trait that has driven me

MY FIRE TRUCK

in everything I do, but mainly in sports and my pursuit of success. Put a problem in front of me, tell me I can't do it, suggest I am incapable of doing it, and you know what? I am going to find a way. I am going to make it work. Say no to me, and I will look for a fire truck and hurtle down that hill.

As I said, I'm not sure where it comes from, but both my mom and dad, who followed careers in healthcare and education, respectively, certainly gave me a degree of determination. Theirs may have been quieter than mine, less showy, but along with my sisters, who have faced their own trials with strength, I can now see it is very likely a genetic thing within all of us.

Neither of my parents are from Florida. My mom, Rhonda, was born in a small town in Alabama called Bessemer. It's so small, in fact, that she tells people she's from the nearby but bigger and more well-known city of Birmingham. While I may tease her sometimes about how small Bessemer is, she always responds with a fiercely protective pride, and she has instilled in me that same love and respect for where I come from. Growing up, I spent a lot of my holidays and summers in Alabama with my grandparents. Barbecuing there on the Fourth of July with my grandad is a powerful memory, so the place feels very much part of my own story.

But my family ended up in Florida because my father, Bruce, had roots there. Born and initially raised in Buffalo, New York, his parents moved the family to Daytona Beach when he was fairly young, and like my mom, he always speaks fondly of where he was born, while also being proud of Florida, a state with so much more to it than just palm trees.

My dad got his undergraduate degree and played basketball at Bethune-Cookman College (now University) in Florida, but went to Alabama to get his master's at Tuskegee University. It was there he met my mom, who was studying in her freshman year and would be the first person in her family to graduate from college. They later got married and settled in Tallahassee, where I was born, and because of my dad's job at Florida State, our family lived on campus.

Tallahassee is not very well known outside of Florida. It may be the state capital, but when people think of Florida, their minds tend to go to Miami, Orlando or even Tampa. For me, though, it is still home. I may have traveled and lived all over the United States, but returning to Tallahassee always feels special. Those early years spent in the dorm still feel so fresh. A small apartment – a living room, two bedrooms, a small kitchen and a bathroom, all on the ground floor – and above us, just concrete and hundreds of students.

When I was four, we were joined by my sister, Laurel. And it wasn't long before the family moved from that world of mine, buying a home in Tallahassee's more affluent Northside. There, in a larger house, we welcomed Eleana, my baby sister, and it was in this home, in what was considered a more privileged, predominantly white neighborhood, we all grew up.

I was a happy kid. Always smiling, polite, but also hyperactive and sometimes overly aggressive. I had a will to win, a desire to battle, to make it work, to find a way. On the sports field, that passion was clear from an early age. The staff at my elementary school, also on the Northside, noticed this about me right away.

One evening, my mom and dad attended a parent-teacher conference, and while my report was a good one, the teacher informed my parents that I was very active, and during recess I was prone to playing "too hard". That description brought a smile to my father's face. "He's not in trouble, right?" he asked. I wasn't.

"So, what do you want me to do about it?" he asked. "He's competitive, he plays hard, he wants to win. I can't and won't change that."

My dad saw something in me from an early age, the same thing that my teacher had noticed: a streak in me that wanted to win. While he had worked hard to earn the money for a nice house and life in Tallahassee's Northside, he knew that if I was to succeed in sports, playing among the children my age and in that community wasn't going to challenge me sufficiently.

So, my athletic life took place on the Southside, a predominantly African American part of town, literally on the other side of the train tracks that run through Tallahassee. My dad decided that not only would I play there, but I'd also be playing up. With that teacher's words in his mind, *He plays too hard*, he wanted me competing against older and bigger opponents.

He felt that I needed to be challenged, that my competitive spirit needed harnessing. It was strange playing with and against kids I didn't know, and being hit on the football field by older and, frankly, much bigger opponents felt different –

hurt, even. But I could compete. I learned that to solve any problem on the field, it was okay to fail. Fail, fail again, but learn. Soon I began to figure things out, and I started to get stronger and better.

As I began to excel at sports, I needed the same challenge in the classroom. I was not extremely interested in academics. I needed to be pushed. A teacher needed to pique my interest, make learning relevant to me. If they just told me to go to school and be a good student, that wouldn't be enough. But if they told me to earn good grades because then I could play more sports, then I was listening.

It was the same in class. I responded to teachers rather than subjects. A teacher who showed an interest in me, making me feel cared for and important to them, would get my attention and hard work. They couldn't just tell me I was wrong, they had to tell me why. They didn't have to be overly nice to me, just honest and truthful, and then they had my attention.

I discovered that I could draw and excelled in art, and I loved writing. I also liked public speaking. I wasn't the smartest in class or overly confident, but I had things to say and enjoyed saying them. In math, I struggled. It wasn't the teacher's fault, but I got frustrated. On the field I loved problem-solving – playing quarterback requires, in many ways, a mathematic mind – but at school I allowed myself to get frustrated and get it wrong. That's why, when playing football, however hard the situation became, frustration was an emotion I always strived to suppress.

In the last year of middle school, frustration came to me for other reasons. We were teenagers, and all those curiosities you have as a teenager were beginning to bubble to the surface. The problem I had, or felt I had, was that there were big cultural differences between my dad and the parents of the kids I went to school with.

Parties were an issue. Even in middle school, kids in seventh and eighth grade were into drinking, taking drugs and smoking. Parties were regularly thrown, but my hopes of going to one were regularly thrown out the window. I couldn't figure out why.

My classmates' parents would go out of town, and my friends would have parties – it even felt like they were encouraged to. I would hear all the stories at school. You can imagine why I wanted to be there. I was a social kid; plus, there would be girls there, and this was a chance to hang out with them outside of school.

"No." It was always a flat no from my dad. No conversation, no opportunity to reason with him. "No." I would retreat to my bedroom, thinking he was my nemesis, an enemy determined to ruin any chance of fun I may have. But Dad was aware what went on at these things, and his son wasn't getting involved.

Now, the thing is, if my parents (and this was the same in many other Black families) ever went away for the weekend, they were taking me with them. It was as simple as that. Leaving me in the house while they were away to do as I please? Well, that was not an idea that would ever be entertained. To my parents, the film *Home Alone* was not a comedy – it was a horror.

Even if I wanted to go to a friend's house, there would be questions. Simple but effective questions.

"Dad, I'm going to Billy's house tonight."

"Oh, that's nice," he'd say. "Just tell Billy to call us and have his parents tell us what time to drop you off and pick you up."

A long pause.

"Oh, Billy's parents aren't going to be there."

"Well, okay then, you're not going."

And that was the end of the conversation.

It wasn't that my parents didn't trust me, it was just how they were raised, and how they wanted to raise us. I was young, I was curious – very curious – and while I might not have gotten into any trouble, theirs was a safe method of parenting, one that knew about the real world and tried to protect me from it.

There were, though, plenty of chances to get into trouble at school and during sports. Playing sports in a different part of town – a, let's say, rougher part of town – and then going to school where I did, meant that kids made their minds up about me early. Too early. At football on the Southside, I had proven myself to my teammates, but our opponents would think I was soft, an overly privileged kid not able to look after himself when things got tough. At school on the Northside, some kids, maybe because I didn't go to those parties, felt that I was overly protected at home.

MY FIRE TRUCK

They all underestimated me. Yes, I am polite. Yes, I seem like a gentle soul. But in my mind, when pushed, I am the undisputed heavyweight champion of the world. By being on both sides of the so-called tracks – playing football on one and living on the other – I had a brawl on my hands in two different environments. But the outcome was going to be the same: I was going to fight my way out of any problem put in front of me.

I used my fists as a way of making the person picking the fight realize that starting it was fine, that was their right, but I was going to finish it. I never started one, but I never, ever ran from a confrontation. I was relatively small – something I overcame on the sports field – but I had a strong mind and body, and as with most setbacks in my life, I was going to find a way. If a bigger kid tried to intimidate me or block my path, then it was on.

When high school came around, these problems continued to present themselves, especially in my sporting life, which was becoming more and more serious for me. Those making the decisions about my football career, and which position I should play, were proving to be frustrating. What I wanted wasn't what I was getting. But here's the thing: What those people didn't know was that, in my heart, I still had that fire truck.

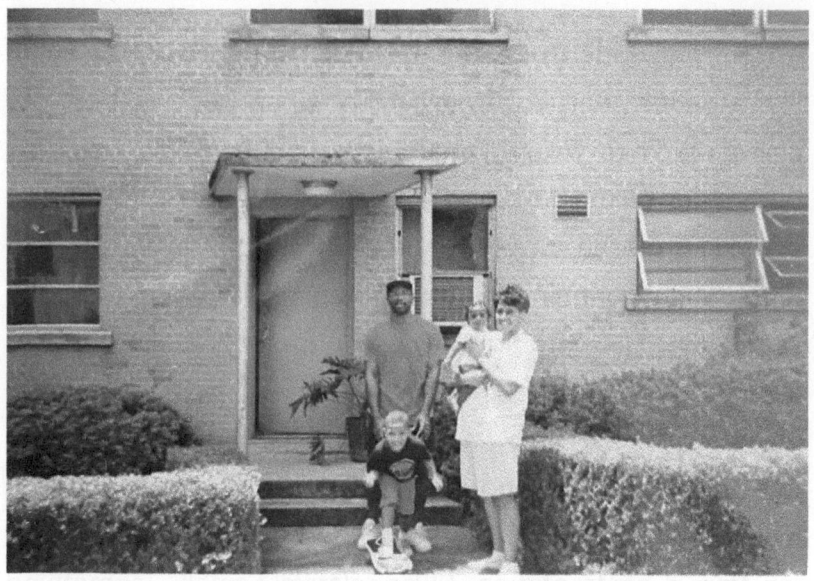

Me, my family and my skateboard

3

I'M SHORT, I'M BLACK, I'M A QUARTERBACK

REJECTING STEREOTYPES AND FINDING MY PLACE

3

The line of scrimmage. Moments from chaos. Thoughts run through my head as, just yards away from me, there are men who want to break it. There they stand, ready. What are they planning to do? Hurt me, prevent me from moving my team forward, destroy me. The play is set, I start the snap count… I can hear those men, grunting, baring teeth, chomping to get through my offensive line and at me. "Hut… Hut… Hut!" It's on.

CRASH. The sound of metal on metal. CRASH. Pad on pad. CRASH. Muscle on muscle. The world around me flies by at a million miles an hour. But then the ball is in my hands, and everything slows. That ball feels right there, everything feels right. I look up, I know my play, I see my receiver, and in slow motion, I bend my arm, snap it forward, and the ball is released into the night air. Life is good.

***

Throughout my young life, sports always made life good. I cannot remember a time when sports weren't on my mind, when I wasn't at my happiest with some sort of ball in my hands. Moving, running, trying to score, trying to be the best on the court or the field – it seemed that this was the place where I could be at my happiest, where I could slow down the mayhem and chaos of everyday life and just be myself.

I wouldn't say that sports were the be all, end all of my family's way of living, but they did play a big part in who I was. As I said, my parents worked in education and healthcare. Hard work was the key to everything, and I certainly understood that that ethic had to be utilized in sports too, but genetically, there was athletic prowess ingrained in my DNA.

My father played college basketball, and my mom ran track in high school. My uncle, Paul Daniels, was a college basketball player at Auburn University in Alabama, where he played with Charles Barkley, who, to this day, remains a family friend. So, sports were always there, literally in the room with us at all times.

As soon as I could walk, there was a basketball for me to play with. I can't remember, of course, but there are photos of me, a ball and a small hoop my father put up. There I am, dunking the ball, a smile on my face, determination in my eyes, and undoubtedly loving that feeling that only sports can give me.

Outside of my genetics and living-room hoop dreams, sports were everywhere. On the campus at Florida State, the football players seemed superhuman. I would be playing outside of our apartment, and they'd go strolling past in their team tracksuits. They had a certain swagger, as if they knew something that the rest of us didn't. From that young age, I wanted in on the secret.

I'M SHORT, I'M BLACK, I'M A QUARTERBACK

When I was very young, the college's star player – in both football and basketball – was Charlie Ward. As I grew up and watched his NBA career flourish, I marveled at how he had played two sports on the campus where I lived. A Heisman Trophy winner, he led the FSU football team to their first-ever National Championship in 1993. I was only three when that happened, but his name and achievements were spoken of so highly that he became a symbol of what could be achieved.

He was a quarterback, he was not the tallest of men, and he was Black. My mind was made up: Charlie Ward would be my role model. Although he went pro in basketball rather football, his shining example was a beacon for my own athletic ambitions.

Apart from his achievements and his ability in both sports, Ward had a way about him. At FSU, playing quarterback, he was determined to be among the first picked in the NFL draft. He wasn't, so he changed course. Despite being a relatively small 6-foot-2, Ward was chosen to play point guard for the New York Knicks. There was a defiance to him, a "do it my way or not at all" that I loved and respected.

I think his attitude was something that I took into my career, through school, into college and then into the NFL. My talent was in the quarterback position. That was where I belonged, amid that chaos, with the ball in my hand, life in slow motion. Others who made decisions felt that wasn't my place. They thought I had no right to be there. "You, a quarterback?" they'd ask with disbelief, looking me up and down.

"No," they'd say, their minds made up. "I don't think so."

They had certain traits in mind, traits they felt were mandatory when it came to playing in the position that I knew was mine. "You're not a certain weight," or, "You're not 6-foot-plus," and this one, just implied: "You're not white." It was always there. A stigma surrounding the position and who played there, a player who would undoubtedly become the face of the organization. An eyebrow was always raised, and too often it was followed with a "no".

The thing is, I wasn't that kid who took "no" as gospel. In fact, I was the kid who heard "no" and interpreted it as "try harder". As a kid, if someone told me not to touch the stove, I would ask, "Why?" They'd tell me, "Because it's very hot," and I would ask, "How hot?" and try to touch it. As a kid, I had lots of Band-Aids on.

As a young football player, those Band-Aids were replaced by a fierce determination to prove myself. I was fighting every day. Fighting the doubts and battling against the stigma that surrounded Black quarterbacks. Huge strides – thanks to people like Charlie Ward – have been made, but as I was growing up, those doubts were very much there.

As a quarterback, you're the face of the program, so they want to know, are you smart enough, can you be trusted with the responsibility? Yes, I was an awesome athlete, but at quarterback, as the heartbeat of the whole team, there were always doubts.

My size was always another issue. As I grew up, becoming a young man, I stood at 5-foot-11, under 6 feet tall, and therefore deemed too small for the job. There is a valid argument for a quarterback having to be at least this height. You are, after all, standing behind your offensive line – the center is usually the size of a small building – and you need to be able to see over them. They couldn't tell me I was too small, though. I was an athlete, and I would make it work. That was my thought process, anyway.

It always had been. I've never liked soccer, but put me on a soccer field, and I will try to score goal after goal. It's a very individual way of thinking, one that I tried to harness as a kid. However, it took a lesson from my dad at a young age to realize the importance of a team ethic.

When I played basketball at about five years old, I had a similar problem as the one I have if I'm ever on a soccer field: I would not pass the ball. I would not look at where my teammates were. I probably felt that I was the best, so why pass? We'd score if I had the ball, so I'd keep it, dribble it, shoot and score the points.

One day we played a game, and I spent the entire first half not passing. The opposition's coach, she knew what I was like, so she told her players to guard me. She didn't want BJ Daniels to beat them on his own. So, all five of the players were on me, surrounding me, frustrating me, making me cry. I was getting so mad, but still I tried to dribble and score all the points myself.

At halftime, with tears running down my cheeks, my dad took me outside and into his parked car. He told me, "Son, if you want to be great, there are certain things you have to go through. If you want to be amazing, you have to use the people around you."

I was only five, but those words really got to me, and I have never forgotten them. I can't tell you what happened in that second half – I'd like to think I passed our way to victory – but I do know that my dad's words, and the intense way in which he said them, stuck.

My dad always knew how I operated. If teachers said, "He plays too hard," he was happy to hear it, and having played college sports, I think he saw something in me that suggested I had what it took to be successful in sports, too. Sometimes, my drive and desire to prove people wrong frustrated him. When we played catch in the yard, I would purposefully overthrow the ball, to show him how good my arm was getting. He'd stand back, I'd carry on trying to throw it over him, or even over the wall in our backyard. The looks he would give me wouldn't stop me, either. I had a point to prove.

He was my dad, but I had something I wanted him to know: I was the best quarterback around. At elementary school, Dad coached my football team, and he would not play me where I wanted to be. He knew I was the best in the position, but he wasn't going to budge because he felt that the other parents would think I was getting special treatment. He thought that if he played me there, I'd be seen as the coach's son with the coach's son's privileges. Plus, he thought I served the team better in other positions.

It was hard. I was young, but it was my first experience of the frustrations that would follow me throughout my athletic career. "Play me at quarterback!" "No." I now understand his reasons, and that he was fending off the other parents' negativity, but being asked to play in running positions, such as receiver, "due to my athleticism," was a line that later stuck.

Unfortunately, as I grew and went into middle school, the same frustrations came with me. Once again, as I tried out for the football team, it was clear that I was the best quarterback. I'm not saying that in a conceited way; it was just that I knew football, I very much backed my ability, and I could see that others going for the same position weren't as good as I was. "Play me at quarterback!" "No." There it was again. The coach (for the first time, not my dad), had seen me play, and there was that line again: "Your athletic ability will be better served in running positions."

For so long, Black quarterbacks suffered from stereotypes regarding our athleticism. Utilized so often in positions such as running back and wide receiver, it was easy to think that our coaches felt that we couldn't be trusted to play at quarterback, even if it was so blatantly our best position.

So, I spent middle school playing football, but not wholly enjoying it. Despite not playing at quarterback, I never confronted the coach, never tried to disrupt things. People would tell me that even Michael Jordan got cut from a school basketball team, and that greatness would always find a way. Maybe that made Jordan a bit more human, but when you're in it and you're young, it's hard to keep your cool. The thing is, I knew that quarterback was where I belonged, so I continued to work on my game, knowing, hoping, that one day a coach would do the right thing. For now, my middle school coach would not budge, but neither would I.

Things would be different in high school, wouldn't they? That's where I'd get my chance, right? I thought so, but then I heard who was coming with me to high school to coach the junior varsity team, and it seemed my hopes would, once again, be dashed.

4

THE OTHER SIDE OF THE TRACKS

GROWING THROUGH SPORTS AND BECOMING MY OWN MAN

4

The green football field, brightened to that lime color by the stadium's floodlights, ushering in the night's entertainment. I loved playing high school football, and I adored playing in college. At high school, there was an excitement to those Friday nights, the whole community coming together, and I had an eagerness to show my peers what I was capable of. And then I went to college and started living for Saturday games, getting out there with my teammates, a group that becomes your world, representing a school that meant so much to so many people.

It was all about enjoying the moment, something not always possible in the pros. In college, for example, you spend the entire week around your teammates – you go out to eat with them, you sleep in the same dorm rooms as they do, you go out to party with them, you practice with them, every day, and no matter what, you know that they will be your teammates that whole year.

It started in the summer. There we all were, alone on the campus, training, getting to know each other, pushing our ambitions, making friends for life. On the weekends we would travel from Tampa to the beach, where that camaraderie would continue to be built and honed.

In the NFL, it's a lot more like a revolving door. With guys getting cut every day, there is a constant insecurity hanging over so many on the roster, making it hard to settle and harder to get to know the guy next to you. The NFL is real life, it's difficult, there is a lot to think about and get wrong, but as a kid playing in high school, and then as a young man at college, we played with a childlike, carefree attitude.

We played the game a little looser in high school and even college. Less tactical than pro football. There is no surprise in that. There, in the NFL, it is the best of the best. Everyone playing is at the highest level. But that's not how it is in college. Not everyone is on a scholarship – you have walk-on guys, seniors playing with freshman, everyone doing their thing, but all trying to win the game with a fast-paced fun. I loved it. I loved how expansive it was. The spread offense. A little more run-and-gun.

We were carefree. None of us were dealing with life's issues. There were no bills to pay, just people taking care of us, making sure we all had what we needed to succeed. The world was ours in the safety of our college cocoon. It was the best, but as I left middle school for high school, 13 and hoping to at last show my small world what I could do as a quarterback, I had no idea of the good times to come. Instead, like most teenagers, I was only worried and concerned for what would come next for me.

When I left middle school, the football coach there, a man who had refused to play me in the position I wanted most, came with me to coach junior varsity at my high school. It was a huge blow. He had made it very clear throughout my time on his team that I was not suitable to play quarterback. Instead, he had me in the "athletic" positions, at wide receiver or running back. "That's where players like you do best."

They were words that hung over me like a gray cloud. I carried them with a sadness that, at that age, I found hard to explain. My strong arm, my on-field intelligence, and the fact that I had consistently tried to show how much knowledge I had for the role of quarterback – none of it mattered. I wanted to escape, so high school couldn't come quick enough. But then the news came that this man who had passed judgment on me was coming along too. I thought to myself, *I guess I'm not playing quarterback, then.*

But then, a switch flipped inside me, just like it did when I turned my fire truck into a skateboard. I knew I had to find a way, to make my ambitions work. So, instead of trying out for that coach's junior varsity squad, I went straight for varsity tryouts, and I performed so well, I was chosen to play quarterback.

I was thrilled. I had proven so many people wrong. It felt like I was changing the world. Of course, I wasn't, but in my mind, I had taken a huge step to prove how good I was. The coach hadn't deemed me good enough to play at quarterback for him in middle school, but here I was in high school, just 13 years old, and I was good enough to play varsity with kids 5 years older than me. How could I not think those negative decisions had not been personal? How could I not think they were based on things other than ability?

Today, I can look back at that time in my life not with resentment, but with pride. Not only for the athletic ability

I showed, but more importantly, for the drive in me to make it work. If I could meet that coach again, I would buy him dinner. I mean that. I would buy him dinner, and I would tell him what his actions did for me. By making assumptions about me, he spoke to a relentlessness inside of me, and for that, I would sincerely thank him.

His actions, my response to them – it was all a valuable learning experience that I would need to remember in other key moments in my career and life. I have a strong faith in God, and I thank Him for allowing me to draw on these experiences and use them as a tool to face whatever challenge may lie around the corner.

For now, though, what was around my corner was high school, and after earning that spot on the varsity team, it was a corner I couldn't wait to turn. Lincoln High School in Tallahassee seemed like the center of the whole universe, a huge place where the freshmen had to learn quickly how to swim… or face sinking.

I was lucky. I had football. By playing sports against kids older than me for so many years, I had become immune to the nerves that I am sure my peers felt about being the youngest students in school. Football prepared me for so much. Looking back, I truly had no fear. Moving through those new hallways, an experience that should have been intimidating, I had no concerns.

What I know in hindsight was that I also had a certain level of inexperience and immaturity. It allowed me to move from situation to situation with no fear, living purely in the moment. Being just 13 and playing varsity didn't faze me because of how I grew up, and how I always played with kids who were older than me anyway. I wanted to be a successful high school football player, and if that meant competing with and against the city's best and brightest, then so be it.

You could say I had a healthy disrespect for position or authority. It's another thing I have taken into my adult life. I don't care for status or rank. I take people at face value; I care about how they treat people at all levels. I don't care if you are the President of the United States – my opinion will be formed by your character, how you carry yourself and the respect you show others.

So, even from that young age, and thanks largely to my dad's insistence that I play with older kids, I was more concerned about how a person played against me – I wanted them to show who they were on the field. I'd think to myself, *You're a senior? Okay, but can you compete against me?*

I wonder what the older kids thought about me. I was a confident kid, but I'd be lying if I said being the varsity quarterback at a school that had historically been so successful didn't come with pressure. In terms of football, this was no ordinary school. Lincoln was arguably the best high school team in the state of Florida, winning multiple championships and producing plenty of all-Americans, players who went on to big colleges and the NFL.

That past success was very much ingrained in the school – as players, we were certainly aware of its many achievements – but I tried to take it all in stride. I was one of only two players in the school's history to start as a freshman, and while that mean living up to a lot of expectation, I knew I could handle it.

The team was so good. We played one of the toughest schedules in the state, traveling on the road to schools in Alabama, Georgia and all over Florida itself, and in my four years there, our record in the city of Tallahassee was incredible. In all that time, we lost just one game to another school in the city, and in my whole high school career, we lost maybe eight games in total.

Friday nights were the most exciting night of the week. They were crazy – I feel the same fondness looking back now as I did then. High school games saw the whole community come together, so I always knew that there were people in the stands who went to my church, people who worked at the same hospital as my mom, and community leaders. I also knew that I was going out to play against, and hopefully beat, their kids.

Being so young in varsity, I was aware that people would be watching me and judging me, thinking, *He's too young. He doesn't know what he's doing.* But I loved it. Being the underdog fit with my personality. Finding a way, showing people that their first impressions were way off – I thrived off that, so the thrill of throwing a touchdown pass came not only from what it meant to the team and the game, but also from the fact that I knew I had changed perceptions of me, both in the crowd and among my opponents.

It was about showing people that I had earned my spot on the team, and then, using all my competitive spirit, making sure I kept it. They were great times, playing quarterback, throwing touchdowns, being part of a winning team – it was everything. I played basketball, baseball too, and I ran track, and I loved them all. But there was nothing like Friday night football.

They were nights that came with a certain excitement. Before high school, I had played football to win, learning as I went, fighting to make a point, but now, at Lincoln, the games came with a sprinkle of glitter, and a level of admiration in the school hallways and the community that I immediately liked. Who wouldn't?

I would get home after games and rush to turn on the local news, just to see even fleeting clips of the action. I would then rip open the next morning's papers in the hope that perhaps the sports pages would mention me – and hopefully a winning performance. It was attention that any athlete will admit to enjoying. The roar of the crowd is a lightning bolt, boosting your physicality and ability, pushing you forward, and those years with the school and the community vocally behind me certainly fueled my hunger to play at a higher level.

I have mentioned that I had always dreamed about becoming an NFL player, but they were just dreams. Initially, I just wanted to play quarterback, which I did, and then I wanted to be the reason for my school's success, which I was. But as the years passed at Lincoln, thoughts and motivations turned to the future – and that's when things got hard.

Being out there, playing, that remained my focus and my joy, but with the success that came with winning games and championships, it began to dawn on me that I wasn't getting the same attention from colleges as my teammates. The receivers catching my throws and the running backs gaining yardage with my handoffs, *they* were being watched and ultimately recruited by big schools all over the country: Texas, Florida State and Southern California.

Before, when I was a freshman and then a sophomore, that was totally fine. Those guys were seniors, it was their time, but as I got older and was part of the school's success, I won't lie, I had high expectations that I, too, would be recruited by the bigger schools as well. Going into my senior year, however, I only received two offers of a full scholarship: one from East Carolina University, and the other from the University of South Florida.

Once again, other colleges and their head coaches had a perception of me and suggested I was better off playing with them at other positions. Once again, a slap in the face: those outdated perceptions about both me and playing quarterback in general. I was a senior, I did everything asked of me, I had proven myself as a quality quarterback, but just like those years in middle school, I felt that what I could do with a football in my hands was being overlooked in favor of what I felt were very dusty and unfair opinions about Black quarterbacks.

Unlike those middle school experiences, where I had to rely on my drive and talent, this felt bigger and scarier. I didn't know what my future looked like. For the first time in my life, I sensed that everyone was passing me by. There was frustration and there was anger, and my dad could see that I was far from happy.

He sat me down and we discussed my emotions, and he had me write down all my goals. He reiterated that I should solely focus on the things I could control: my focus, my work ethic, my game, my grades. The politics within the system couldn't cloud any of that. It was a vital piece of advice and, with that, I continued to play well, and my future became less uncertain.

Initially, choosing the right college wasn't easy. FSU was the place I had grown up, the team I had watched with my dad and adored. It was the team Charlie Ward had starred on. But their coaches never offered me a spot on their team.

It was a huge blow, as was listening to other college coaches who I felt showed a level of arrogance when discussing me, my abilities and my physical attributes, which were different than the typical quarterback. They also talked a lot about the success of their programs: *they* had achieved this, *they* had done that. I wanted to hear about how we would work and how we could achieve things together. But then I met Jim Leavitt at USF, and his actions as a man as well as a coach could not have been more affirming.

In my first year at Lincoln, I was the back-up quarterback, as I sat behind senior Keeley Dorsey. Early on in that first season, Keeley wasn't playing well, so after just three games, they brought me in as quarterback, and tried him in a new position.

Keeley moved to running back without complaining. He showed no resentment, just continued playing hard and well, and because it was his senior year, he knew he had an opportunity to progress. Due to his performances that year and in that position, he got a full scholarship to South Florida. We were all so happy for him. He had treated me with such respect, there had been no jealousy on his part, no bitterness, and I was excited to see what he might achieve in college.

And then came the news. In early 2007, during a summer training camp with USF, Keeley had a seizure and passed away. His death shocked the high school – he had been such a big part of our team, and we had taken pride in all of his achievements. His funeral was packed with friends and loved ones, and it was there that I saw a man who was so much more than just a football coach.

Jim Leavitt, Keeley's coach at USF, chartered three or four buses from Tampa to Tallahassee, bringing the entire college football program to pay their respects. His assistant coaches, the staff, the players, the cheerleaders – they were all there. And when Jim spoke, I heard a man speaking out of love and compassion for one of his players, but more importantly, it was clear that he saw him as so much more. He saw Keeley as a young man.

As a high school kid at that funeral, with big decisions looming on my horizon, I was struck by Jim's sincerity. We later talked about me coming to USF, playing quarterback there, the things we would all strive for. Together. Coach was extremely genuine, and you could tell he cared about his players. That sense I had watching him speak at the funeral remained, and I knew that this was the coach and the school for me.

In my freshman year at USF, I got a tattoo on my arm that says, "Live life today. Yesterday is gone, and tomorrow may never come." Keeley had the same tattoo on his back. They were words that seemed so momentous, and by having them on me, I wanted to finish what Keeley started. They remain very important to me now.

Leaving home for college is a huge moment in any young person's life. I was very close to my mom, my dad and both my sisters. Our home, it was all I knew, and like most teenagers, I guess you could say I was more than a little dependent on my mom for the everyday things in life. Fortunately for me (maybe not so much for my mom), I was going to a school far enough away to experience real independence for the first time, but also close enough to visit, and yes, that did mean getting some laundry done and eating some good home-cooked meals.

Living in a dorm, getting to know so many new people, partying: my first year of college was lit. I joined a fraternity, made some mistakes and took on college life with energy. I redshirted my freshman year because the team already had a starting quarterback, and I could maintain four years of college eligibility if I sat out a season. This gave me more time to focus on another sport that USF had recruited me to play: basketball.

Although I was so focused on football, I had continued to play, love and excel at basketball throughout high school – so much so that I had been voted the best basketball and football player in the Big Bend area of north Florida's panhandle, the first kid in Tallahassee to have that honor. I had opportunities to play college basketball too. In fact, as a basketball player, I got a lot more attention from bigger schools than USF. Schools such as Memphis, who had reached the NCAA Tournament Championship game in 2008, were very interested, but my passion for football and my desire to play quarterback were too strong to ignore.

For now, though, I was on the court rather than the football field. I planned to focus on football after my redshirt freshman year, and while basketball came with less pressure, it didn't come without its issues, and once again they involved myself and the coach.

We didn't get along. We had very different visions and ideas about how I should be doing things on the court. I was young, I was confident, but I felt that confidence was backed up by my talent. My coach didn't see it that way. When it came to the star of his team, he had someone else in mind. That was never going to be easy for me to hear.

I knew the guy who my coach favored. Everything on offense had to go through him. However, I had played against him in high school, and in those games, I felt I had been the better player. After all, I competed against him, took him on, averaged around 27 points a game in high school and won that vote over him for the Mr. Basketball award in my area. The confidence that came with all that didn't like being quashed, and yet, there we were with everything being set up for him to be the star on the court.

I can look back today and admit that I could have been more humble, less vocal in my disapproval. It was the perfect storm of youthful ambition meeting unchecked ego. I can admit that now, but I wouldn't change it. It drove me, it proved that I had a fire in me. When I was just five, my dad had instilled in me the importance of using and being part of my team, and I had never forgotten that, but that wouldn't dampen my individuality.

Further fueling my ego was the response from the fans, both at USF and opposing colleges. We would go and play in Pittsburgh and West Virginia, and as far away as that, fans would be mocking me, drawing signs, making fun of me for not playing all the time. I had earned a reputation as a good player in both sports, and now I wasn't starting in either.

It was the same at our college. I had arrived with big expectations as a football player, an important quarterback, and yet, there I was, playing basketball – and playing second fiddle to another guy. "Put BJ in the game!" someone would shout from the stands, and the more those words were ignored, the more frustrated I got.

Today I work with students, and plenty come to me with grievances similar to mine: they disagree with a coach, or they feel they aren't getting enough game time. Now, with age and experience, I can, while never diminishing their self-confidence, tell them to do everything they can to figure out how to get on that court or field.

I tell them to fight but not to complain too much. I was vocal in my frustrations to the coach, but I eventually realized that to get where I wanted to be, out there playing, I had to understand the politics, be smart, play my role. I've had coaches try to belittle me in a room of my teammates and peers. They would ask me all sorts of questions about the game, setting traps to embarrass me. They wanted to make it clear, simply from a knowledge standpoint, I was not ready to play.

But then, I would fight fire with fire. I learned quickly that athletic ability isn't enough. To truly excel, it takes more than being in the gym and out on the practice field. So, I'd go away, learn that playbook like my life depended on it. Not only would I force them to notice me and my ability with the ball, but any question they tried to bamboozle me with, I would have the answer. Try to take me down mentally? Well, I'd be prepared for that too.

The good thing was, I was learning all these life lessons and soon, they would benefit me out where I most wanted to be: the football field. After playing just two games in my redshirt year, I returned fully focused on my first year on the football team.

Maybe there were still some doubts about my ability, my stature and my knowledge, but I felt sharp. I was the back-up quarterback, but in the first three games, the coach put me in for a few minutes, and I quickly confirmed that I could do the job on the college level. When were playing Wofford from South Carolina, I threw a touchdown pass, and it felt so good.

In that moment, the opposing defense did something unexpected, I improvised, and because of that, the play had opened up, and I could throw the touchdown pass. It was a special moment. Nothing big in the history of college football or even USF's highlight reel, but for me, that thought process, taking hold of the moment with my mind as well as my body – well, from then on, I knew that I could be a success.

That was the mindset, but then it was a waiting game, and the key to it all was being ready for my chance to prove it.

THE OTHER SIDE OF THE TRACKS

I was the back-up quarterback to one of the greatest in USF history, Matt Grothe. Matt was a star, but I put everything into my work and trained like I was starting every week. Chances come, and there was no way I was not going to be ready if the opportunity presented itself for me to touch the field.

I worked out harder than ever, I ran harder in practice, sprinting from end zone to end zone, doing extra weights, putting in extra practice alone, watching films, studying the playbook over and over. In my mind, I had to be the main man. After voicing my frustrations at not being the star of the basketball team the year before, I knew that now, silently, without any attitude, I was just going to be ready to show it.

Sometimes, when you're young, it is easier to get mad at what you see as the injustice of your situation. Friends, family, the fans, the media – they are all full of questions about why it isn't working out for you, but you have to shut all that out. Keep your focus. I realized that quickly, so my focus shifted onto working harder. After that, everything seemed to happen so fast.

The thing about sports is that one man's gain is usually another man's disaster. Three games into the regular season, Matt Grothe tore his ACL. Of course I felt bad for him, but then my mind cleared away that sentiment because I realized that, next week, it would be my turn to play. And the next week's opponents? Florida State, of course.

Florida State, the college that had rejected me, and now, I was, for the first time, starting as quarterback – and playing against them. The thought of what was to come could have gotten to my head. The chance, there in front of me, was a chance to show the FSU doubters what they had missed out on. The temptation, at the back of my mind, was to make the game all about me.

But instead, I felt very different. Calm. The night before the game, I was in the hotel with the team, and my mom and dad came to visit. It wasn't long before my dad noticed that difference. I had a strange expression on my face, like I was deep in thought.

"What's up, son?" he said.

"We're gonna win."

It was as simple as that. It scared my dad how at peace I was with what was about to happen, how sure I was of what was to come. It was like I said, as a kid, when people told me not to touch the stove, I wanted to know how hot it could be. At FSU, too many people had told me no, and now I wanted to bring that same heat.

The next day, we were at the Doak Campbell Stadium in Tallahassee. We were warming up out on the field, and I was doing some stretches alone. Then, Coach Leavitt came over to me, and he saw tears rolling down my face.

"What's wrong, BJ?" he asked.

"I'm okay, Coach."

"Why are you crying?"

"Coach, I am sitting on this field, and I'm looking up at the exact seats that me and my dad would sit in together, watching Charlie Ward play."

"I get that, BJ," he said, concerned. "But are you okay?"

"Coach, I've never felt better."

In my first-ever start for USF, I went out onto that field and had the game of my life. I passed for 300 yards, the most any quarterback had achieved against Florida, threw two touchdowns, and we left as the winners, 17–7.

17–7. I am a religious man, and in the Bible the number seven means completion. That day, I wore the number seven jersey. That day wasn't about completion – there was so much more to be done – but it was about being there at the heart of my team, in front of my family, my mom and dad's colleagues, old friends from high school, in the town in which I had grown up. It was a personal dream coming true, just not in the way I'd ever dreamed it.

From that day in my hometown, I played the rest of my college career with a smile, the same smile I wore on Friday nights playing high school football. With that came some success, and with success at quarterback, minds began to turn to the future. In the distance, it was possible to see the bright lights of the National Football League.

I'd had dreams before, and some even started to come true. Could they again?

5

SEVENTH ROUND

THE PRESSURE, EXPECTATIONS AND REALITY OF THE NFL DRAFT

It's a spring Saturday lunchtime in 2013. Myself, my family, my girlfriend, her family – we're all sitting in my parent's living room in front of the TV for what is now the third day of the NFL draft. For three days, we have gathered here, waiting and hoping. The balloons they put up have lost their air, and the pizza has gone cold. We're down to the seventh round of the draft, and the name "BJ Daniels" still hasn't appeared on the screen.

My family, my girlfriend and her parents are all putting on brave faces, still trying to muster smiles, but their eyes give them away. This may not happen for me. The dream may not come true. I sit, feeling alone. Their words of encouragement fade into the distance, as I contemplate that I may not make it. All that effort, all that hard work, all the extra practice – maybe it wasn't enough.

Suddenly, I'm scared. Fear. What now? How do I face so many people who believed in me? What do I say to all the people who will try to be polite? How will I look into so many eyes and see such disappointment? Fear.

But then, I think back to just a few years before, and I try to make sense of what I have been through. Fear? It hasn't been that long since I discovered the true meaning of the word.

***

It was my sophomore year. Thanksgiving. I was attending a party thrown by the rapper Plies. He and I were good friends. Plies is from Fort Myers, not far from Tampa, and after that win against Florida State in my freshman year, I got a lot of attention from a lot of people. I received a new amount of admiration and fame in the area, so when Plies approached me, we hit it off and struck up a friendship.

So, that Thanksgiving, he was throwing this party. In a strip club. A rapper's party in a strip club. I laughed when I thought back to those middle school parties that my dad wouldn't let me attend, because they would have been tame compared to this. But I was a young man, at college, living independently, making my own decisions. So, I decided to go. I didn't tell my mom and dad though. Some things never change.

Anyway, I was at this party with three of my college teammates. We all listened to and liked Plies's music, so it was exciting to be invited. I had suddenly become a recognizable face, Plies was obviously recognizable too, and we were all living our best lives. I'm not going to lie, it was a lot of fun.

We partied into the night, staying longer than even Plies. He left, but my teammates and I were enjoying our minor celebrity status too much to go home. We were going to stay as long as we could – maybe a little too long.

At around 4am, we finally decided to leave. I was the designated driver for the night, and I had left my vehicle behind the club in a dark parking lot. My teammates and I walked toward the car. I was at the front, with my three teammates ten feet behind me. I could hear them – we were

SEVENTH ROUND

all laughing about the night we'd just had – but then I turned a corner, caught sight of my car, and the laughter stopped. All I could hear were footsteps, and they were running.

I turned around, wondering what was going on, and I came face to face with a gun, held by a guy wearing a ski mask. Around him were three other guys, also in ski masks. At that point, I had dealt with a lot in my life, faced opponents on the football field and gotten into so many fights with guys much bigger than me. But I had never felt fear like I felt right then.

I instantly saw the white light – yes, the one everyone tells you about, it's a real thing. I dropped to the ground – I'm not even sure if they told me to do that – and something inside of me simply said, "Survive." So, I started emptying my pockets. I threw my keys, I threw my phone, and as I did, I couldn't hear or see anything, probably from a combination of adrenaline and fear.

Then, I felt something cold on the back of my neck – the barrel of the gun that had been in my face just seconds before. I took that as a signal that they wanted my necklace, so I ripped that off and threw it, too. Only then did I hear something: the sound of the masked men running off into the darkness.

Then, silence.

I was all alone. The white light disappeared. There was just darkness. I felt around in the dirt and found my phone, and then I lifted myself up and headed back into the club.

It was a life-changing moment – one that remains with me today, and one that affirmed the mantra that I have tattooed on me, that you have to live for now. You don't know, sometimes literally, what or who is around the next corner. As a 21-year-old, it dawned on me again that life is too precious to take for granted.

Back in the club, I told the security guards what happened. Some of them were armed and went outside to investigate, but there was no sign of anyone. They asked about my teammates, and I was distraught, worried that the masked men might have found them, and they were now dead on some sidewalk. I kept calling them, but there was no answer. Eventually I got through to one of them, but he did not want to tell me where he was. He thought I was setting them up, that the guys who robbed me wanted to find out his location. That's how scared he was. He didn't come back to the club at all.

One of my teammates had his brother come pick him up, and the other eventually came back to the club from his hiding spot. I was able to locate my keys once it was light out – remember, I threw them while I was emptying my pockets – and at 6am, I drove home, showered, put on a T-shirt and shorts, and went to a team meeting at 8am. Two hours later, I was at practice. Running on only adrenaline.

I may have been in state of shock, but I wanted to continue with my day. I didn't call the police because I didn't want it be in the news. I could already hear it: "BJ Daniels, starting quarterback at USF, robbed at gunpoint!" I didn't want that. I didn't want the coaches at USF or the school to know. It happened, and I wanted that to be the end of it. I didn't tell Plies, either. I didn't want him to have any link to what happened. I knew the media might get ahold of it and just

SEVENTH ROUND

see it as a rapper's birthday party that got violent, playing into all kinds of stereotypes. I didn't even tell my parents. I just wanted it to simply go away. It happened, though, and I couldn't suppress it. So, since then, I have tried to use the intense fear that I felt that night in my everyday life.

At practice the morning after the robbery, there were my teammates, the ones I had been with the night before. Now, you might want to know, was I mad with them for running away? The answer to that is no. I put myself in their shoes, and having experienced the same fear as they did, I knew why they ran. I didn't run, even though I wanted to, because I had recently suffered a blood clot in my thigh after a hard hit in a recent game. Running, for me, had not been an option, but I understood their instincts and I couldn't be mad.

A couple of years later, sitting on my parents' couch, watching the draft, three days in and still waiting for my turn that didn't look like it was coming, I felt fear. There was no sudden blindness, no falling to the ground, and certainly no bright white light, but, and as much as that incident outside of that club had forced me to look at life from a new perspective, I couldn't shy away from the fact that my future seemed uncertain, and I was genuinely scared.

Just two days before, the room was full of hope. On Thursday, the day of the draft, my parents set everything up. The living room looked great: balloons were hung, and the pizzas and chicken wings were out. It was all there, and being with my family, my girlfriend and her family, it really felt like a celebration.

For me, though, that party spirit had already, even on that first day, disappeared. I didn't want to bring the atmosphere down, but when it's your future on the line, it's hard to pop bottles too soon. What the people in the room didn't know was, even on that first day, I was already feeling anxious. I felt like I had already missed out.

I was in the NFL draft. On one level, that was a childhood dream come true. But I wanted more. That's the competitive spirit in me. I wanted more, and that meant not just being in the draft, but being invited to the draft. On that first day, I looked at the guys, about 50 of them, invited to New York, to the NFL headquarters for the big TV reveal, and I watched as they were called up on stage, wearing suits and knowing their families were in the crowd, not at home on the couch.

I busted my ankle toward the end of the college season, and could not make the televised tryout, the NFL Scouting Combine. I couldn't even play in either the Senior Bowl all-star game or the pro-day tryouts, and so I was left on the sidelines looking in, hoping that my efforts through my college years would give me enough of a chance.

The injury was a big blow to me, and on top of that, the season with USF had been frustrating. We weren't successful, and as captain of the team with big ambitions, I really felt that failure. I wanted so much. I wanted to be a National Championship winner, I wanted to be the Heisman Trophy winner, I wanted to be healthy and get a real shot at the dream. None of these things had happened, so while on draft day there were smiles, expectations, the smell of good food, and the clinking of glasses all around me, I was worried.

SEVENTH ROUND

All the doubts crept back. My height, my broken ankle, the fact that I am Black; would an NFL team take a chance on me at quarterback? Could I trust my agent, a man I had only just met and hired to work on my behalf to sell me as a quarterback? Was he saying the right things, the things I had told him about my desire to play at quarterback, or was he simply thinking about dollar signs and, no matter the position, selling me to the highest bidder?

My phone kept buzzing. My agent was sending texts and making calls, telling me that the Eagles might be interested, then nothing. "Might be"? What did that mean? Another call, this time it was the Giants who could be interested in signing me. Too many doubts. Too many possibilities. Not enough certainties.

Next to me, trying to be supportive, was my girlfriend. However, we both knew that our relationship was becoming just as uncertain as my future. We had met when we were just 15, while I was playing basketball against her high school. We were together ever since – she even went to USF – but things hadn't been easy.

I can admit that becoming a success as a freshman football player at USF changed me, and I didn't handle what came with my newfound fame as well as I could have. I cheated on her with another girl. We tried to work through it, but things were rocky. On top of that, sitting next to her on draft day were her parents. Now, I had no idea what they thought of me, and I had no idea if she had ever come home to them in tears, telling the truth about me and our relationship. It added to the tense atmosphere, as did the fact that we were with my two baby sisters, my two biggest fans who probably had their own thoughts about whether this girl was good enough for their big brother.

Thursday, the first day of the draft, came and went. Then Friday. Still nothing. Saturday morning, and everyone was still in the room. Their support meant so much to me, but that morning was the hardest. It was Saturday or not at all, and with the stress, doubts and fears, I thought back to my college career. Could I allow myself to let those doubts win? Could I start to think that it was all for nothing?

Playing college football, as I have said, those were probably the best days of my life. On a good day, playing in front of 75,000 fans in a sold-out stadium in Tampa, throwing touchdowns to my teammates, playing against the biggest schools, such as Notre Dame, Florida State and Miami – it was unreal.

Just after the armed robbery outside of that club, in my sophomore year, our team was preparing to play a bowl game, essentially our championship game, at the end of the season. I had that blood clot in my leg, so it was uncertain if I'd play, but I was desperate to take on Clemson. They were known as being one of the top football programs in the country, far better than us, and we were very much underdogs going into the game. But that was fine.

Before the game, with the injury, the coaches were unsure about me. Was the leg okay? I was a game-time decision. By then, the head coach at USF was a man named Skip Holts, who had replaced Jim Leavitt that previous summer. Jim had total faith in me, but now, Coach Holts had doubts and put me in a quarterback competition with a guy who was a walk-on. He had no scholarship, while I did, and I'd already played my part in beating other teams, big teams, and somehow, I had to fight for my place in the starting line-up. I was pissed off.

It was a huge blow to my ego. I was already frustrated, and then the injury meant I couldn't compete to the best of my ability and show the coach he was wrong. The fact that I had to once again prove myself enraged me, but he was a new coach, so I knew I'd have to do it again. From the start, I didn't think that Coach Holts believed in me in the same way Jim Leavitt and the university itself believed in me. So, him forcing me into direct competition with the back-up quarterback was another blow to our relationship, and with the biggest game of the year in front of us, the potential for him to not play me was a frightening one.

Fortunately, I proved to the coach and his medical staff that my leg was okay, and Holts put me in to start. But in the third play of the game, I threw an interception. An interception! Maybe the coach was right. That was that, I thought. I didn't convince the coach. He saw the game differently from me, he seemed ready to replace me, and then, immediately, I gave up possession. I fully expected to be taken out of the game.

But then, he didn't. To Skip Holts's credit, he gave me another shot at it, and from there, my team and I soared. We won the game 31–26, and I was named MVP. It had been a crazy few weeks: the robbery at gunpoint, the injury that might have cost me my place in the biggest game of the year, those doubts from our new coach. No one really knew how intense it had been because I held it all in. So, after the game, when I was asked to come up on stage as MVP and say a few words, I kept it simple.

"How do you feel?" I was asked in front of 75,000 people.

"I thank God," I calmly said. "I'm thankful to be here, I'm grateful for the opportunity, and this means more to me than you'll ever know."

With that, I left the stage. I was grateful to be there, to be alive. I was grateful to the coach for giving me the opportunity. It was a case of trying to figure things out, making things work, even in the face of adversity, and there on the stage, my simple message to the crowd and those watching on the television summed that up.

Those were the big moments, and with them came more and more attention. In the stands, there was so much passion for what the team was doing from the people, the community who came to games and took such pride in the school that they, their parents, their grandparents, and maybe even their children went to. That came from both sides. Playing on the road, in front of hostile crowds who felt as passionately for their college as USF fans did ours, I loved every minute of it. You can argue that college football is far bigger, in Florida and across the South, than pro sports, and playing in that environment, competing and excelling, it was like nothing else.

Soon, it became clear that NFL teams were watching and the draft was a very real goal. Going into my senior year, that was the only thing on my mind. It was time to fully prove myself as a quarterback. I'd seen players, very good players, drop their levels in their senior years due to the

SEVENTH ROUND

pressures that come with the knowledge that scouts were watching them. Judging them.

Each game you play is an audition, and I was determined to catch the scouts' eyes, every week. All my focus was on what I needed to do. Of course I wanted to make the team successful, but in my senior year, this was it. I had to get *me* right, work harder, make certain that I was handling my business the right way. Do all that I had to do to get noticed.

I wasn't alone. On the USF team, there were five of us getting attention from NFL teams, and we became a team within a team. Holding each other accountable. Never letting standards slack. If one of us wasn't putting in what was required, the other four would rally around him. All five of us had come to college together, and now all five of us were pushing each other to take the next step.

Two of us were on offense, the other three were on defense, but it didn't matter: That year was about a togetherness that I'll never forget. The team itself, though, that was less focused. In short, my senior year, the team wasn't very good. Winning games became very hard, and with such big goals ahead of some of us, that was hard to take. A lot of the team lacked both ability and ambition, but I couldn't resent anyone for that. It was just how it was that year.

There were frustrations. Of course there were. As the quarterback, I wanted to be throwing game-winning touchdowns, running game-winning yards, but that wasn't happening. But I was the team captain, so I certainly wasn't going to start bringing down my teammates or blaming them for not playing at a certain level. We only won three games that season, and there would be only eight quarterback picks available in the draft, but I had to have faith – faith in my God and my work ethic – that what I was doing was enough.

All five of us NFL hopefuls had that desire, that faith, in ourselves and in one another. Today, over a decade later, we are still in touch, still watching out for what the others are doing. All of them made it into the NFL, and now all of them have made their lives successful. One owns a crane company, one has a couple of restaurants. It's a privilege to know all of them.

But I didn't know that as I sat in my parents' living room, the clock ticking on the last day of the draft. My possible career was at the forefront of my mind. After breaking my ankle and missing the last games of the season, the thought of being overlooked wasn't a new one. In terms of what I might do next, my mind was on the degree I had gained in criminology. I had already been on a police ride-along, and a possible goal was joining the force before ultimately joining the FBI.

The FBI? Maybe that was where my ambitions should lie? In terms of football, as that clock ticked, it became clear that I was not on any most-wanted list, and you didn't have to be a special agent to see that my mood and hope had both gone dark. Those around me continued to be upbeat. "Not long now, BJ," they'd say, but I was hardly listening. I was thinking about all those who thought I would make it, all the people I thought I was letting down. It didn't make sense, but I felt like I'd failed.

And then my phone rang.

SEVENTH ROUND

It was a number I didn't recognize. My agent hadn't been in touch with any word of offers, so I wasn't expecting any teams to call, but I stood up to take it anyway. I walked out of the room just as I heard a voice on the other end of the phone. "Hello, it's Jim Harbaugh from the San Francisco 49ers."

Quickly, I was in my parents' bathroom. The door was locked behind me. For some reason, I wanted to be alone. I thought that it could still be bad news. I was pleased to hear his voice, but other coaches had spoken to me, and nothing had come of it. So, I locked myself in the bathroom in case it wasn't the news I wanted – that way, I didn't have to look in my family's eyes while I received it.

"How are you doing, BJ?"

"Coach, I'm not going to lie to you. I'm frustrated."

"Are you healthy?" he asked, knowing full well that I had suffered my ankle injury.

"I'll tell you this," I said. "I'm well enough to make the 49ers a better football team."

That was that. He told me there and then that he was taking me to San Francisco. I was an NFL player. It happened so fast. We said our goodbyes, and I stood, taking a second, looking at myself in the bathroom mirror. It happened, and now it was time to go out and tell my...

Before I could turn the lock, my mom was screaming at the door and practically beating it down. She and everyone else had seen my name come up on the TV screen. Before calling me, Harbaugh had already told the NFL of his intentions to sign me, and so, it was official.

To the sound of my mother's screams, I opened the door and was hit by a wave of love. My mom grabbed me, she held me close, and I began to sob. I couldn't stop. It was a release of years of trying. It was a release from everything I had kept in. Being held at gunpoint, the frustrations from elementary school to college, of not being trusted at quarterback, to proving people I should be. It was a release from the pain of the broken bones and clotted veins. It was a release from the very real knowledge and fear that sometimes, however hard you work, dreams don't come true. But mine did.

I stood in my mom's arms and sobbed like a kid. Real tears. My mom held me, and she wouldn't let me go. My parents had nurtured me, they'd nurtured my competitive spirit, seen my ambition and given me all the support they could to help me make that ambition happen. Now, as the emotion poured out of us, my mom stood and supported me once again.

Soon, everyone was with me, the anxiety that had filled the room was gone, as if a window had been opened, and fresh air filled every corner of the house. I could breathe easy. At last. As the news began to get out, the phone started to ring, calls from people I knew well, calls from people I didn't know well, calls from people I did not know at all. It had happened. I was going to the NFL.

It would take days for the reality to sink in, though. Plans had to be made. I was heading to California, to San Francisco, to the 49ers, one of the most iconic names in our game. I was heading west and, like the prospectors in 1849, I packed my things and hoped to find my fortune when I got there. Soon, though, I would discover that not all that glitters is gold.

6

A DREAM COME TRUE... KIND OF

THE STRUGGLE TO STAY ON TOP

6

"How did you know?"

It was the only question I could think to ask. As I stood, alone in an airport in Tampa, on what should have been the first day of the rest of my life, my head was instead full of doubts. Doubts about myself, doubts about what my employers would feel about their new recruit, and doubts about a future that just hours before had seemed full of possibilities and hope.

It was two weeks after the draft, and I was on my way to Rookie Mini Camp in San Francisco, the first opportunity for the new draft picks to get together. We would be joined by guys trying out for the team, but not the veterans, certainly not Colin Kaepernick – just us rookies and members of the practice squad who had played minimal or no pro football. So, I headed off to the Golden Gate City, but more importantly to the NFL, and that morning's flight was supposed to get me right where I wanted to be.

I missed it.

I missed the flight. To this day, I cannot explain why or how I missed that plane. My time management was off, I was unprofessional, and there was no excuse. A psychoanalyst might argue there was a deeper reason, and they might be right. I might have had some reservations about taking the steps to leave the state that had always been home, but as I stood in that departure lounge wondering what my next move was, I was sure that by missing it, my character was going to face immediate questions.

It should have been the most exhilarating time of my life, but I knew I would be heading into an environment where people would look at me and say, "There goes BJ Daniels. He doesn't respect people and their time."

While I was checking out my options, looking up at departure boards, asking about connecting flights to San Francisco, embarrassed and desperate to get moving, my cell rang. For the second time in two weeks, it was the 49ers head coach, Jim Harbaugh.

It had been just 30 minutes since I had missed the flight. Just half an hour, and I had not yet told a soul what happened. Unlike our first phone call at my parents' home, this time, Coach Harbaugh's voice was not a happy one. "You must think this is a game?" he said.

I was shocked. More embarrassment washed over me, but as I stood there, all I could think of to ask was, "How did you know?"

There was a pause. And then Coach said something I'll never forget. "We are a billion-dollar industry. Why would you think I wouldn't know?"

It wasn't as if I needed a reminder about the size of what I was getting into. The sheer size of both the San Francisco 49ers and the NFL in which they played, but Harbaugh's words floored me. When he then said, "You must not want

A DREAM COME TRUE... KIND OF

to be here," the realization that I'd jeopardized not only my dream but the way people saw me, well, that broke me. There in the airport, I began to cry.

Through my immaturity and inability to get prepared, I harmed myself and my chances. I had, I presumed, also let down someone who had always done his best to progress my ambitions. Jim Leavitt, my coach at USF, the reason I choose the school, the coach who had faith in me to play the way I wanted to play, he was now linebacker coach at San Francisco, and it was a pretty good bet that he would have vouched for me before Harbaugh's decision to draft me.

Eventually I got another flight, but as we rose above the clouds, a dark one hung over me, and as we landed in my new home, I was very aware that I had a lot of work to do. Perhaps more than most. When you make a mistake like I did, the first thing you want to do is get in there and make up for it. I was going to be even more polite than I usually was, make every curfew, be the very best version of myself; I was going to somehow make an extra effort on and off the practice field, but I knew it was a battle that I might never win.

At the back of everyone's mind – or so I feared – would be the fact that I arrived late. However polite I was, *I didn't have the manners to get there on time*. However hard-working I was at practice, *I didn't have the work ethic to make sure I was on that plane*. You want to be on time, polite, nice, answer all the questions, but inside you know that no one really cares. Deep down, you know that everyone knows you're the guy who missed his flight.

Luckily, there was a glimmer of hope. In the NFL there's something called "The Giant Eraser". It's a joke within the game, one that I hoped would help me. Basically, it means that the mistakes made by players throughout the week can be erased by what they do on a Sunday. Let's say a player doesn't perform well in practice on a Wednesday, but come Sunday, he is the best running back in town, and whatever happens before that was forgotten. And that is even truer for the quarterback, who always has to be on time and on top of his game, setting the example and leading the team.

So, I missed my flight, and I also hadn't made the cut yet, but I wanted to, so it was a case of getting to Mini Camp, working hard, then working harder. I knew people might say, "There goes the guy who missed his flight, he must not be taking this seriously," but I had to make sure that, soon, that changed to, "That guy can really throw a football, he's definitely taking this seriously."

I arrived in San Francisco and got to work. To walk into the training complex and be around people who wanted exactly what I wanted, it hit me that *this* was the pro game, and I was now in it. I was part of it, and every day I wanted more. The thing was, as we went to work at the rookie camp, there were no feelings of closure. I did not go to bed at night thinking, *That's it, I made it.* Being in a professional football environment only added fuel to the fire of my ambition.

Leaving Florida, people that I grew up with might have said goodbye to me while thinking, *That's that, he did it, BJ is living his dream.* But the dream was never to just make the NFL, the dream was to play in the NFL, and there, in that camp, I knew and respected the work that still had to go into making it. Even today, when I meet people and they find out that I was involved in three Super Bowls, that I am friendly with Odell Beckham, that's what they want to talk about. I don't blame them. I get that the big moments that come with a pro career can seem more appealing than the everyday hard work, but the struggle, being cut, waiting as the backup and waiting some more, that was my truth, that's what gave me the battle scars that have shaped me. It was all about the struggle to play.

Of course, not everyone saw it that way. As I said, after I was drafted, in many people's eyes, people very familiar to me, my dream had come true. I made it. My life was set up, the checks were big and they were regular, and from then until the end of my life, things would be plated with gold.

It happened immediately. In college, I used to get my hair cut by a friend. The guy was from Tallahassee, we knew each other from our high school days, and knowing that I had no money, he helped me out. And then, days after the draft, I walked in, we chatted, he did my hair, I stood up, went to shake his hand, and he said, "That'll be $40."

Now, I am not complaining about my friend trying to earn a living, and I wasn't expecting free haircuts for the rest of my life, but the speed of that change and how it came immediately after the draft opened my eyes to the fact that perceptions and expectations of me had radically changed overnight. BJ Daniels was no longer a college student trying to make ends meet; he was a superstar athlete with money to burn.

Suddenly, it also dawned on me that the cocoon that life with my parents afforded me, and that college gave me, was gone. I was on my own and I had stuff to figure out. That shouldn't have concerned me. I had spent my entire athletic career to that point trying to do just that. Quarterbacks figure things out, right?

Get the play, know the play, see the play and execute it. Simple. But life, as I learned very quickly after moving to California, doesn't play out in the same way it does on the field. If only. As a young man, fresh out of college, I was comfortable on the field. Big guys trying to hit me – I could handle that. A clever side step, or a change of pace, and they were gone. But out in the real world, where agents, banks, real estate agents, and even relatives and friends wanted to take a bite out of your new fame, those side steps were harder to find.

Great uncles and cousins that I didn't know I had, acquaintances from my hometown, were suddenly very much in my life. Could I hang out with them, could they borrow some money? There had to be a bank account brimming with cash now, right?

Fortunately, the family members close to me, those who had seen my efforts over the years, knew the truth. They also knew that none of this had been motivated by wealth. My mom, my dad, my sisters – today all four of them are in service-led careers. My dad is a professor and event coordinator at an HBCU (Historically Black Colleges and Universities), Florida A&M University, and has been a girls' high school basketball coach for more than 15 years. My mom has been a nurse for more than 35 years. My sister Laurel is a third-grade teacher, and my sister Eleana is at the University of New Orleans, where she is director of player development with the school's women's basketball program.

While my ambitions were always in sports, and yes, a benefit of being in the NFL was the money, it certainly wasn't why I wanted to be there. My family members who watched me sweat, bleed and prove people wrong for that dream, they knew the truth – I just wanted to play the game.

Initially, my mom and dad flew out to San Francisco with me. I was hunting for an apartment and felt I could use their wisdom. And there I was, after all, fresh out of college with no credit to my name, but I was being shown very expensive condos. I didn't really have a clue what I was doing, and there was so much to adjust to.

I waited to bring my girlfriend out. I wanted to be on the team's playing roster before she made the trip, and that was going to take hard work and concentration. Once I settled into practice and began to work as hard as I could to make people see me as the athlete I knew I could be, the scale of the task in front of me was daunting, but I knew I could do it.

I was working through that ankle injury from my senior year at USF and getting stronger, but I was also up against five other quarterbacks on the team, and one of them was Colin Kaepernick, one of the best in the world, who guided the team to the Super Bowl the year before I arrived. On top of that, I had to learn a new language.

An NFL playbook makes the college version look like an elementary school brochure. It was thick as a dictionary and sometimes so dense it seemed like another language, and I had two days to learn it, but I somehow did it. Football is all about communication, and it's vital that you know how to communicate with your specific teammates, so nearly every hour without the pads on, I had my face in that book, learning how the team would talk, making sure I was fluent in what made the 49ers tick.

I quickly realized that one of the most important and lauded components on any football team was the quarterback, and in San Francisco, that man was Kaepernick, a player who possessed an abundance of ability, personality and belief. Colin was the heartbeat of the team, and I knew that while he was not going to be budged in terms of me being more than his backup, I could learn so much from him.

It was a strange dynamic. A rookie like me arrived, eager to get started, desperate to prove myself, and Colin was there, established, focused on his performances, but also willing and happy to help me. Just not too much.

We were living with different pressures. Mine stemmed from being noticed, getting onto the team. Colin, on the other hand, knew that, like anyone else on the team, he was just one injury away from losing his job. At any moment, for example, he could've fractured a pinky finger, and he'd have to sit it out for three weeks. In that three weeks, BJ Daniels, the rookie backup, could step in and do a great job, help the team win some games. After that, Colin would possibly be viewed as injury-prone, maybe a bit soft, and then there would be a whisper that maybe it was time for a change on the roster. Colin would come back from injury, throw a bad first pass. An interception. People would whisper, "Are his mechanics gone? Does the team miss the rookie?" With all that in mind, the likes of Colin Kaepernick can be friendly, and they can be helpful – and he was – but they're never going to just let someone take their spot.

I understood that. I understood the game. So, what I did was give absolutely everything on the practice field. Players like Colin had Sunday or Monday night to think about. They would practice knowing to leave plenty in the tank for game day. Not me. I was trying to get noticed Tuesday through Friday, and that meant giving everything, every time.

Practice was my playground, where I wanted the staff and my new teammates to see the very best version of me. Whether I was playing receiver, running back or with special teams, what I put in was going to be my all. Running, throwing, learning, everything I was doing and offering was 110 percent, and with that came an initial recognition.

In August 2013, in one preseason matchup against the Kansas City Chiefs, I got on late in the third quarter, threw six completions out of nine attempts, led all the team's quarterbacks by throwing 72 passing yards and running 13 yards, and I delivered the team's game-winning touchdown pass.

After the game, Coach Harbaugh was asked about me and my efforts. "Going into what he did the other night, it was very positive," he told the Associated Press. "It was an encouraging performance, and he's done some encouraging things in practice as well. So, he continues on his process, and he competed well and made plays. And when somebody does a good job, you give them a little more."[1]

That little more was a place on the team. Suited up for the start of the NFL season. It was a huge boost. I wasn't guaranteed much playing time, but to be part of the 53-man active roster, proved to me that, despite the letdown of missing that flight, my hard work and attitude had in fact changed some perceptions.

I thought I was finally getting closer to my NFL dream. I just had to keep doing what I was doing. Keep working, proving that I belonged there, and good things would follow. I believed that, but then I learned that in the NFL, I never stood on solid ground – it was more like thin ice. And it wasn't long before it began to crack under my feet.

It happened one morning. I showed up at the practice facility, and I was standing in the locker room when he started to walk toward me. Who do I mean by "he"? Well, each team had one, and we called him "The Grim Reaper". Nothing odd to look at, not old, not flashy, but he wasn't our friend. He was just the guy who, if he talked to us, it usually meant bad news, and if he said, like he did to me, "The coach wants to see you upstairs," it meant, nine times out of ten, we were in big trouble, or worse, we were about to get cut.

"The coach wants to see you upstairs." That sentence hung in the air. "Get up there and bring your iPad and playbook." I knew that meant he was probably going to ask

A DREAM COME TRUE... KIND OF

me to hand them in. So, I headed up those stairs, wondering why, after all my hard work, the Reaper had chosen to visit. And when I walked into Coach Harbaugh's office, I could tell that all those fears were justified.

The coach stood and told me that they had their eyes on another quarterback, that he was off the street, meaning a free agent, and that I was going to be cut so they could take a closer look at him. I stood in silence. There was no point in vocalizing my inner anger, which came from not being given the chance to compete against this guy.

That was all I did since I'd arrived: compete. And I competed hard enough to learn the playbook, hard enough to always be on time, hard enough to catch the coach's eye in practice and the preseason games, and hard enough to make the initial list of 53 players. Now, without a chance to fight, I was being told, in an office, that I was being cut to the practice squad.

NFL rules state that, for 24 hours, a player has to sit on the waiver wire, a database for all free agents, and if no one picks you up or you decide not to move when that 24 hours is up, you stay with your team, but on their practice squad. That meant no chance of playing.

It was a huge blow. Financially alone, the hit was a big one. On the active roster, I was earning a minimum of $22,000 a week. On the practice squad, that would drop to about $7,000. Of course, to so many, that is still good money; I understand that. Regardless, that wasn't the biggest blow – it was how I was seen by the team.

The respect with which the team held me dropped like a stone. On the practice squad, I was there to make up numbers, service the team. Having experienced the opportunities given to those on the active roster, I wanted to be on their level once again. I was so disappointed by the decision, but I knew that the decision was made. No amount of protest was going to change any minds, and as angry as I was, I could look in the mirror and be happy with what I saw looking back at me. I had arrived on the other side of the country, and I had done everything in my power to make it work.

The following day, I had until noon before my time on the waiver came to an end. By 11:30am, it looked like it would be the practice squad for me. Then, my phone rang. It was Pete Carroll from the Seattle Seahawks, and he didn't waste any time. "BJ, we only have 30 minutes. How do you feel about becoming a Seahawk?"

I was mad at the 49ers. I had done all I could, and without so much as that chance to compete, they had dropped me. I also knew that very few people on the waiver list had teams come in for them, and there I was, being approached by another top team on the West Coast. I would be crazy to turn them down. "I feel good about that, Coach," I said. And with that, the deal was done, and I had to report to practice in Seattle the very next day. That's how quickly lives in the NFL get turned upside down – all it takes is a 30-second phone call.

Without even saying goodbye to my teammates, I packed one bag and headed to the airport. I had ended up renting an apartment in California, but I left it, the rest of my belongings and my car until I had a place in Seattle and could hire movers to bring everything to me (and yes, that meant I had to pay rent in both places for a short time, too). But that wasn't even on my mind – I was on another flight, this time to meet a new coach and a new set of men that I hoped to call teammates. I was as eager as I had ever been to prove people wrong. What I didn't know was that in Seattle, that attitude was going to make me plenty of friends.

7

KEEPING UP WITH THE JONESES

ADAPTING TO CHALLENGES – AND SUCCEEDING

It's the fall of 2023, and I am in Seattle. With my friends.

I am here to mark the tenth anniversary of the Seahawks' Super Bowl triumph and immediately I feel at home. If I spent my career chasing something, my time in Seattle was the closest I got to finding it. It was there that I felt even the slightest sense of permanency, that I felt part of something. Among our group of players and staff, there was a unity that I cherished and will never forget. It was a feeling that I felt cover me like a blanket (very useful in this cold and wet part of the world), while I lived there and as soon as I landed.

There is an energy to Seattle. An energy that links its people to its football team, and no other Seattle team has given those people more to scream about. There was plenty for us guys to yell about too. A whole decade had passed since the night we took that huge bite of the Big Apple and brought the Seahawks their first Super Bowl championship.

A whole decade, ten years in which so much had happened to all of us. Careers had gone in different directions, lives were being lived in so many ways, but the moment we all met, coming together again at the stadium where we had shared so many special moments, and it was as if we had never been apart.

There was something unique about this group. We shared so many triumphs, overcame so many obstacles, faced hard times as one, and that connection remained very much alive. Being in the city itself was wonderful too. Like I said, I fed off the energy and, of course, it was inspiring to take part in team signings, where I got to meet thousands of fans within a community that still appreciated me and my efforts. If I'm being honest, as I flew to the Pacific Northwest, that's what was on my mind. *Would the people remember me? Would all the hard work I put in for their team be appreciated?* I wasn't Russell Wilson, but to be there, and to experience the positive reaction, was special.

Special, but, I soon realized, not the most important part of the trip. Sitting and signing autographs, having the people of Seattle greet me with such enthusiasm, that was what I thought I wanted, but then I met and spent time with the mother and sister of one of my closest teammates.

Tarvaris Jackson, or "TJack", as he was affectionately known, was a popular and loved member of the team. Like me, he was a quarterback, although he played for four years in two stints with the Seahawks. He had a ten-year NFL career before retiring and serving as quarterback coach at Tennessee State University. In the spring of 2020, Tarvaris was killed in a one-vehicle car accident, just days before his 37th birthday.

I always liked Tarvaris. Like my mom, he came from Alabama, and working with him as back-up quarterbacks, we gelled and became friends. He often talked about his home and his family, so to be introduced to his mother and sister, who had traveled to Seattle to be there for the reunion, meant so much.

In the ten years that her son had played pro football, Tarvaris's mother, Sasanque, never managed to see him play in Seattle, but she and his sister felt a calling to come from Alabama to Washington and meet the guys who were so proud to know her son and call him a teammate and friend.

I sat with Sasanque, and we talked. We talked about good times, her son's commitment and work ethic, but also his smile, his love of life. She told me that she had heard a lot about me, and those words were very emotional, not only reminding me of the loss we all felt so deeply, but also just how close that group of men were. To hear that Tarvaris had, years later, spoken to his loved ones about me and the group, underlined just how much of a family that Seahawks group had become.

Yes, being in the city, hearing the fans cheer again, being reminded of the glory that we had all experienced was nice, but it was that moment with Tarvaris's family that symbolized what the trip was actually about: people coming together who meant so much to each other and who, through sheer hard work and teamwork, made our dreams come true. Life had moved on for us all, of course, but that season on the Seahawks shaped us all, and as soon as we were together, that feeling of brotherhood was powerful.

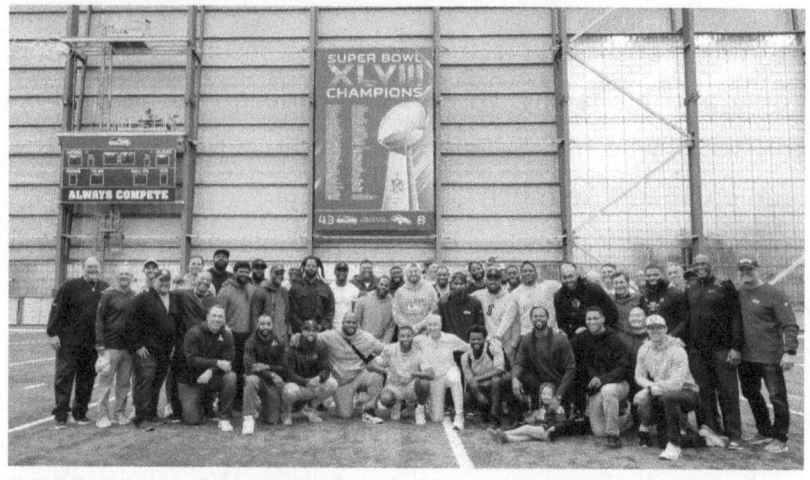

Seahawks reunion, 2023

***

It had happened quickly. I certainly felt it soon after I arrived in Seattle in 2013, a decade prior to that reunion. I was a new guy, I had a playbook to learn and a city to settle in to, as usual, but there was something here that I liked from the get-go. The people here were interested in more than me as a player – there was an interest in how we were as men. They asked about home, college, family. People cared for one another, looked out for the guys next to them, and all those feelings of belonging rushed back as I sat with Tarvaris's mom and sister.

Such unity can only harbor success. Trust me, I have been in locker rooms that offer very little togetherness. A group can be full of talent, packed with guys who individually would break most teams. But if a group has differing goals, if its members aren't together in how they want to achieve those goals, then all the talent in the world means nothing.

I have been in groups where some people were just interested in fame, or they were in direct opposition to the guy sitting next to them who might have taken their place on the starting line-up, and that hadn't gone down well. To be competitive, there has to be a degree of selflessness, of course. You want that spot in the team, but support the guys around you, and only good things will happen. Otherwise, it can get really ugly.

I've seen fights break out. That can happen in even the most solid group. And these are 6-foot-plus, 300-pound men we're talking about. Fights are going to happen. Every guy that I played with fought with someone. No one could be happy all the time, and yes, punches were thrown, benches were tossed, but as long as it came with respect, then that was fine. It was kind of like fighting with siblings. I love my sister, and when we were little, we'd fight; however, I would never allow someone else to hurt her. In a good squad, we might fight, but we also love. And on game day, it was our turn to fight everyone else.

In a weak locker room, those confrontations linger, they simmer, they don't get fully resolved, and when game day comes and you have to fight together as a team, something is always missing. Those cracks turn into holes, and thoughts of success are lost in the darkness of them.

At Seattle, there seemed to only be light. It felt different, and credit for that has to go to the head coach, Pete Carroll. Coach Carroll was different. Coach Harbaugh had been all business at the 49ers, and Coach Carroll was much more relaxed. He was immediately energetic – that family vibe was there from the start.

There was a lot to like about Carroll. He was very laid back, friendly and open. I could see by the way that he treated everyone. From star quarterbacks to the catering staff, he was the same friendly personality. With rookies like me, his closeness was impactful, and I could sense that he was a coach and a man to whom it would be easy to give my loyalty.

He had an ambitious streak that was infectious. His desire to achieve things, to be the best, that was clear, and it wasn't long before I was ready and willing to take the leap with him. What I liked most about Pete Carroll, though, was his sense of optimism. I had, for so long, been used to coaches, from childhood to the NFL, who, frankly, were pessimists. "No" was the easy way out. "That isn't possible." "No way, you can't do that."

Then, I was face to face with this guy. This guy who believes anything is possible, who believes that through sheer belief and teamwork, that tiresome and restrictive "no" can become an affirming and challenging "yes". That's why I believe that the group we had at the Seahawks was special. So many of us had faced the pessimism, we had heard that "no" too many times. We had been told that we didn't fit, but here we were, with a coach who saw things differently. Okay, let's get to work.

I always think of the Seahawks that I played with and think of the word "redemption." We were a redemption team, a team of misfits, and I immediately felt at home.

There I was, this undersized Black quarterback, playing backup to Russell Wilson, a Black QB with a similar stature to mine.

There was also Marshawn Lynch, from the mean streets of Oakland – East Oakland, to be exact. His mother raised him and kept him out of trouble; you could say that football saved his life. His NFL career started with the Buffalo Bills, but he was young, and made some mistakes while he was there, the typical ones that many rookies make. He was traded to the Seahawks after three years in New York, and he was ready to prove himself in Seattle.

We also had Richard Sherman, the corner from South Central Los Angeles, who had two very distinct sides to him. One was the Stanford graduate who is an NFL announcer now, incredibly well-spoken and put-together. But he was a completely different person on the field: aggressive, passionate and loud.

There was also Doug Baldwin, an undrafted free agent who played at wide receiver, written off by so many as too small or too slow. And Kam Chancellor, the safety? At 6-foot-3, many said that he was simply too tall for the position, that his height would affect his mobility, but it turned out he was among the quickest and strongest in the game. On the flip side of that, there was Earl Thomas, a free safety deemed too small for the NFL.

It felt like a mismatched group, we all had something to prove. Pete Carroll himself had come to Seattle in 2010 and shortly after that, he became tarnished with scandals regarding his college players and the improper benefits they received from marketing men and agents. Some pointed out that, though he'd enjoyed an incredible career in the college game, he never won the National Championship. Was he really that good? Yes, Carroll had to work to reclaim his own reputation. He, like all of us, sought redemption.

Everyone was an individual, but our shared experiences added to the sense of brotherhood that, although I was only in San Francisco for a short time, I hadn't felt with the 49ers. The approach there was very different. Jim Harbaugh was a totally different kind of man and coach to Pete Carroll. That's not a criticism – Harbaugh was very successful, but I quickly learned from working with him that his style of management was more of the challenging kind.

I also learned very quickly on the 49ers that being a rookie counted for very little. I was thrown in at the deep end, and there was no life jacket. Walking in and working with the likes of Colin Kaepernick and Anquan Boldin, as well as Harbaugh himself, that was strange. These were superstars, guys I had watched on TV for years, and I won't lie, to suddenly be among them and competing with them was a shock to the system.

And then I had to be their leader. That's what a quarterback is. When I was playing, whether in practice or on game day, I had to make these guys feel they could trust me, that they could follow me, and those early days were spent trying hard to prove myself worthy of that trust.

In the huddle, there is only one voice. It is the quarterback's, calling the plays, directing the offensive line. The quarterback is the coach on the field, and I quickly learned that the reputations or the fame of those I was directing meant nothing. Nothing at all.

My age, my lack of experience, the amount of years I had under my belt, the levels I had been at before – it meant nothing. If I was calling the plays, these guys, some of them Hall of Famers, had to listen and respond, without question. I can't tell you if it was hard for them, but it was a difficult transition for me, made harder by a head coach who, as it turned out, did not have any kind of faith in me or my ability.

Things came to a head fairly quickly. Days prior to our first preseason game in the summer of 2013, Coach Harbaugh asked me to draw up some plays. I was supposed to pick ten of my favorite ones, draw them up on a piece of paper and bring them to the quarterback team meeting. I was still learning the playbook, he understood that, but I went away and enthusiastically got to work.

I then came to the meeting with my thoughts down on paper, interested to get Harbaugh's thoughts. As I was still learning his playbook, I presumed that he wanted to know what plays he could call, plays that I knew and was confident in.

I stood up in front of my teammates and coaches and presented the plays, drawing them up on the board in a clear fashion. I thought things were going well, but then Harbaugh turned. He began to ask questions. He asked me about details on each play that he knew I would not know yet. These were high-level questions, the answers to which I couldn't have possibly known: "What would you do if this play went wrong?" Things like that, when I was still working on the basics.

I knew that the receiver needed to be here, that the running back was going to be there, that the offensive line was blocking certain people, but I didn't know the finer details, so he chose to embarrass me in front of my new peers. I couldn't understand why he would do that. Sure, educate me, help me learn the playbook (something that I was spending every hour trying to do), but don't intentionally humiliate me. Considering that I had missed the plane to San Francisco weeks before, we weren't off to the best start.

He then told me that he wasn't going to play me in that first preseason game. That really pissed me off. Those emotions grew stronger when Harbaugh said he felt that I wasn't taking advantage of my opportunity. I wondered if that had to do with me missing the plane, and that he was going to hold that over me for longer than was reasonable. He must have seen how hard I had been working. Other coaches must have informed him that I was doing all that was asked of me – and more.

I certainly wasn't looking for a pat on the back, but it was a hard time – moving to a new city on the other side of the country, getting through the training camp, dealing with the new media interest, experiencing the physicality of the NFL, learning the playbook, and dealing with a far-from-smooth personal life.

My girlfriend and I had been through a rough patch, and she agreed to stay in Florida until I got settled in California. San Francisco is three hours behind Florida, so, at the beginning, there were late-night phone calls. She wasn't happy that we were apart, and the problems we faced before I left hadn't been completely resolved. We'd talk for hours, late into the night, and I would wake up feeling unrested, so I made a decision.

All my eggs had to go into one football-shaped basket. I needed to dig deep into my mental state, telling myself that this was my dream — that distractions, including my family and my girlfriend, had to be temporarily set aside. So, I lost a bit of contact with everyone. My girlfriend wasn't pleased, but I wanted her to realize that I had to work on making the team, to make a life in San Francisco, one for both of us to eventually share.

They were words that didn't necessarily land on understanding ears, but with my renewed focus came opportunities to play, and in those games, I made sure I got noticed. With touchdown throws and yards gained, I caused a stir with the fans, the media, my own teammates — so much so, that I made the team.

I couldn't work out if Harbaugh was purposefully pressing the right buttons. By doubting me, by vocalizing his concerns about my character and ability, he had created a rage in me, but I had fought on. In those latter preseason games, I might have only had five minutes of playing time, but I was going to get noticed. Put me up against the wall, tell me that it isn't possible, and I am going to make it work.

But, despite it all, the grim reaper still came to San Francisco, and, out of the blue, I was told I had been replaced. Armed, however with the experiences I'd had, even during such a short time at the 49ers, I came to Seattle in a rainy November determined to hit the ground running, and having found a squad of like-minded men, there could be no regrets.

I had learned so much from the 49ers, an elite team, one that made the previous year's Super Bowl, and so when I arrived at the Seahawks, it was with a serious business mentality. I wasn't going to lose my dream again, and so I came with a head-down, "let's get to work" attitude.

And I certainly got more love from Coach Carroll. He reminded me of my coaches from college. Carroll had enjoyed great success at USC and took that style into the NFL. I loved it. He treated us fairly; he didn't have time for berating us or belittling us in front of the rest of the team. Instead, we were made to feel welcome and appreciated.

Don't get me wrong, this wasn't kindergarten. We were there to be pushed, to learn and to compete. It was a tough and intense place to work every day, we all knew what came with the job, but we wanted to do it without being berated and yelled at all the time. We wanted to enjoy the experience. Athletes know they're doing a job, we just don't want it to feel like one. Pete Carroll made sure that was the case.

It began from the very first meeting. Some teams have an initiation ceremony, a new player having to sing or rap in front of his new teammates. But Pete Carroll's initiation was slightly different.

At the Seahawks, there would be a meeting every morning. Everything would be thrashed out. Records set straight. Any problems, any arguments, they were solved there and then. At the beginning of each of these meetings, we would walk in, and Carroll, every time, would have hip-hop blasting from the speakers. Snoop might be on, maybe Drake, and it would be loud. Then, Carroll would walk in, and we would get down to business.

At my first meeting, I was asked by Carroll to come up to the front. The belief behind the Seahawks, the team's mantra, even, was that everybody has a story. It emphasized that fact that everyone had experienced hardship, survived something, that everyone had learned from a negative. "BJ Daniels, come up front and tell us your story."

So, that's what I did. As I was walking up, Coach was underlining things. "This is a loving environment, we all care for each other, everyone can feel free to share their truths." The guys are all hollering and whooping, repeating his words of affirmation. I got to the front, turned to the whole team, Carroll walked up behind me, and slightly nervously, I began to talk.

"My name is BJ Daniels," I said. "I am from Tallahassee, I grew up on the campus of Florida State..." Now, what I didn't know was that behind me, Coach Carroll was holding up his fingers and silently counting down with them. *Three... two... one...* and just as I was about to go into my story, the whole squad stood up and, in unison, shouted, "SHUT UP! SIT DOWN! NO ONE CARES!"

Everyone in the room was hysterically laughing. And there I was, in a vulnerable place, about to tell my story, and the whole room was in on it. It was hilarious and it happened with every new guy. For a few minutes, you were the butt of a very big joke. The moral of the story, though, was that *everyone* had experienced negativity, in the group, we had *all* suffered hardship. It went without saying. You could look at the guy next to you, and while he may have laughed at you during your initiation, you were now his brother.

Like any family, moments like that one brought us together. We became closer when we laughed with each other because it made us realize that no one was bigger than those jokes. It was another case of sharing experiences together. And I immediately felt part of something bigger than a football team.

There was no wondering about anyone's motives. At Seattle, above the door that took us out to the practice field, there was a sign, and every time you walked through it, going out to work, you made sure you touched it. The sign simply said, "ALL IN". And we were.

***

By the time I arrived, toward the end of the regular season, that attitude had gotten the team far. When I got there, the Seahawks were 10–1. "ALL IN." As fate (which seemed to be beside me on every team I played for) would have it, just three weeks after I arrived, we were off to San Francisco.

There were 70,000 people in Candlestick Park that day. San Francisco was so strong at their home stadium, and it was a very competitive game, but the 49ers were the winners, 19–17. I had stood on the sidelines, desperate for some sort of revenge, but mainly I stood and looked across the field, and it was strange to see so many familiar faces.

Not necessarily the faces of Kaepernick or Boldin, but the guys who had arrived with me. Five other young men, drafted together, starting right at the bottom of the totem pole. We lived in the same hotels, and none of us had cars yet, so we'd get rides together. We held each other accountable, pushed each other on, studied the playbook together, making sure we all were on top of it.

These were the guys I had been throwing the ball to. It took weeks before I was able to throw to the team's starting wide receivers, so I practiced with my fellow rookies until I had that chance. Their support was something I'll never forget, and we will all be friends for life. That's why, on that occasion, standing in a different uniform, just months after we had all arrived in California, I was hit with an unexpected sadness. Listen, I was more than happy to be at Seattle among such a great group, but I was the only one who had been cut by the 49ers, and because I hadn't been given any real reasons why, I needed that revenge. Little did I know that I would get a chance very soon.

After clinching the NFC's number-one seed by going 13–1 in the regular season, we beat the New Orleans Saints 23–15 in the first round of the playoffs, setting up a mouth-watering NFC Championship game against, yes, the 49ers. This time they had to come up to our stadium, and what a game it was. I wouldn't play, that was fine, I was still learning the plays, studying extensively after every practice. I admit that it was a lot to take in.

This playbook is given to you, as thick as a dictionary, but one that changes every week, depending on the team you play next. You learn it, and then there's more to learn, and on top of that, the next week's learning is added on top. It's like drinking water through a fire hose.

That's not to say that I didn't enjoy it. Learning not only the playbook, but how to carry myself as an NFL player, was a thrill, one that I loved. And at the same time, I was relaxing into my place in the NFL. There is a rule that stipulates that once you are on the playing roster for a certain number of games, then you cannot get cut. I had gotten through that time limit, so my girlfriend moved out to Washington, and for the playoffs, we gave it a shot, living together as a grown-up couple.

It wouldn't be easy, but neither would that NFC Championship game against our rivals from San Francisco. That's what made it so special. There was and is a very real hatred between the two teams. They are on the same coast and in the same division, so there's a natural competitiveness. But on this day, there were even more tensions because of our personal histories with each other.

The coaches, for starters. Harbaugh and Carroll had enjoyed big battles while they coached at Stanford and USC, respectively. Then, there they both were, coaching at the highest level of football, and it was even more intense. Richard Sherman and Doug Baldwin, players for the Seahawks, were both Stanford players who Harbaugh chose not to take with him to the 49ers, so they were now playing for Carroll. And then there was me and my recent journey from San Francisco up to Seattle.

I was in uniform, and with the best view in the stadium, closely watching a field crammed with talent. Hall of Famers on both sides, a ticket to the Super Bowl for the winners, and in the stands behind me was a laundry list of A-list celebrities.

Actors, rappers, singers, athletes, other football players. Cameras were flashing everywhere – it was like nothing I had ever seen. I thought to myself, *I've made it.*

As a football player, these are the moments you dream of. In fact, they are more than you can ever dream they'll be. I stood there, this huge game unfolding in front of me just yards away, and I thought about my younger self. It occurred to me that, as an ambitious boy, I had never allowed myself to truly believe I would one day be involved in all this. I wanted more, I wanted so much more, but on that day, I could look back at all those missteps, the negative coaches telling me no, the broken ankles, being held at gunpoint – none of it could have prepared me for the joy of being at that game.

And what a game it was. It was arguably the game of the century, perhaps even the best in history. Some experts have called it that. Whatever it was, it was the game that saw Seattle through to Super Bowl XLVIII, winning 23–17 in a thrilling matchup that was a Richard Sherman fingertip away from going the 49ers' way.

After the final whistle, I was able to greet and embrace those friends I had made during my time at San Francisco, but there was no contact, not even eye contact, with Jim Harbaugh. To be honest, even if he had tried to talk to me, I wasn't interested. He had let me go with no explanation, the guy who replaced me had lasted only two weeks, and I had very much moved on. After all, I had bigger things to worry about – the Super Bowl was waiting for us.

***

I remember arriving in New York and looking around at who I was with: a wonderful, irreplaceable bunch of misfits, with venom in their eyes. For the first time since the 1990 Buffalo Bills, we were a Super Bowl team with no Super Bowl experience. Not one of us had been here before, not one of us could draw on his past and understand what was to come, but every single one of us knew what had to be done.

That was very much the team's thought: *Do what has to be done, and glory will follow.* In fact, we weren't concerned about *if* we were going to win, it was always about *how* we were going to win. Go out there, do what we do, execute it properly and we will be victorious. Our attitude was to dominate the Denver Broncos from the first play, but we just didn't expect to dominate them so forcefully.

The way the team began the game, out of the gate at 100mph, was proof of how well the staff had harnessed the anger that was brewing in us all throughout the build-up to the game. We all knew that the Broncos were a great team, and they had great players, but as the days passed, we noticed that the media attention centered solely on them.

The Broncos' quarterback, Peyton Manning, was getting endless attention from the press. It went on and on. I'm not being disrespectful – Peyton Manning *is* one of the greatest players of all time. But as the headlines and commentary continued, we looked around our locker room, and the sense that we had something to prove grew and grew. Soon, we had a new attitude: "What about us? Oh, you don't know about us? Let us show you."

From the first play, the Broncos were steamrolled by that attitude. They were unable to catch their breath. Marshawn Lynch was superb, proving people wrong, and so was Doug Baldwin. Malcolm Smith, another seventh-round draft pick, was rightly the game's MVP.

It was intense to watch the 43–8 victory, and I was so proud of everyone involved. Being on the sidelines, in the uniform, was surreal. There were a several players who I played with at USF on the Broncos roster, something that reminded me of the journey we all go on to get there, but mainly, I was focused on the now.

Russell Wilson was excellent. It's funny. People would ask me, "Do you secretly want him to get injured or play badly so you get your chance?" I can say, hands down, that the answer to both was no. I was ready mentally and physically to play, but I didn't want him to play badly – that would jeopardize our chances to win the football game. Plus, after spending so much time with Russell, there was no way I would wish he'd get injured.

I spent the same amount of preparation time studying the same plays, going to the same meetings and lifting the same weights as Russell. Everything I did was as if I was the starting quarterback, that was my responsibility, and I am very proud of how I carried myself not only during Super Bowl week, but during my entire rookie season.

The Super Bowl ring still gleams when I look at it. Like the memories of the game and my entire rookie season, it shines brighter with time. I was new to all of it, but I quickly experienced the very lofty highs that the game can bring if you and your teammates come together.

"ALL IN." I, however, was about to remember how quickly this game could turn on us, and how some of us would end up ALL *OUT*.

8

"YOU PLAYED WELL TODAY, SON"

HOW PRESSURE AND VALIDATION AFFECT MENTAL HEALTH

8

It's just hours before the first game of my senior year of college. A year that I told myself had to be mine, had to continue building on what I had already accomplished at USF. I did well so far, became a known and respected name in the college game, but I had to keep it up, strive for even more. The NFL was waiting.

Just hours after the game, and that was exactly what I felt I'd done. I'd stepped up. I threw one interception but brushed that off – I picked myself up and kept going, and then I threw three touchdown passes. We won the game by 30 points. The noise of the crowd – those cheers rang in my ears. I could still feel the pats on my back from my teammates, and the words of encouragement from my ecstatic coach stayed with me. At least, they did for a while.

Just hours after the game, I got into my mom and dad's car. To make things even better, they'd made the trip to Tampa to see the game, and just like when I was a kid, I got in the car (riding shotgun) with them after it ended. I relished their words of approval too. Those were simpler times, growing up. Playing football, trying my best, doing well, then sitting in the car and hearing my mom or my dad say, "You did well today, son."

On this occasion, before they could say anything, I turned on the car radio. "South Florida win by 30 points... BJ Daniels throws three touchdowns." Nice. That's the thing. Athletes, we seek validation – no, we *crave* validation. It might start with parents and that "you played well today, son," but it escalates. Coaches, teachers, classmates, the crowd, newspaper reporters, television and radio reporters, and today, the whole world on social media.

That night, in the car, listening to the radio, I thought I had my validation. But then, it happened. On the radio, an "expert" came on and started talking about me and my game. The interception. Nothing about the touchdowns, or the win – it was all about that one intercepted pass. That one mistake. He said how disappointed he was with me, that he thought I'd stopped throwing such passes, that I should have been much better than that, and how my game hadn't matured enough in four years for an NFL opportunity.

His words hit me hard. Silence. After all the night's glory, after all the good things I'd done, one person's pessimism took all of that away. One person felt the need to highlight the one mistake I made, and that was that. The night was ruined.

That night, sitting in that car, I cracked. My parents tried to console me, as usual finding strong words. They told me that if I was going to have a career in sports, I couldn't seek approval from outsiders, and there would be so many voices – to focus on the negative ones would be a waste of time and energy. I agreed, but truth be told, those words on the radio stayed with me, like they would with most athletes.

"YOU PLAYED WELL TODAY, SON"

I've seen it: Pro football players would come off the field, go into the locker room, and the first thing they'd do was check their phones, check to see what the world was saying about them. Looking for that "you played well today, son" that their moms and dads used to give them. These were highly paid athletes. Men seemingly with everything – the clothes, the homes, the car and the money. But they wanted more, and part of that desire was simple: They wanted to be loved.

So, before they did anything, they got on their phones, they saw what the world was saying. If they played badly, would they be the next big joke? Were they the latest meme? My parents were so right when they said that you can't let all the outside voices in, but it is easier said than done, and even the biggest, most successful football player is susceptible to letting those voices get louder and louder. And eventually the noise can take its toll.

Being a pro athlete is wonderful. It's the dream. To spend every day in practice, getting better at a sport you love, to be part of a team, to have teammates you would run through walls for, to go out there every week and to play in front of tens of thousands of people. There is no denying the glory and fame, but there is a price, and sometimes the pressure that comes with the constant striving for success, and that never-ending search for validation, well, it all takes its toll. I saw it, and I felt it.

Social media. Today, it's an everyday part of all our lives. Opinions, photos, videos and some more opinions. They are all out there for the world to see, but when I was playing,

I felt that the noise on these platforms was far louder and far more destructive than any reporter or sportscaster's opinion could be.

Those first doubts crept in back in college. It was my sophomore year, and I had been out with my fraternity, Kappa Alpha Psi, on a Friday night. Then, my roommate called me unexpectedly to tell me that another guy who lived with us had gotten into a motorcycle accident. I was shocked, concerned and very upset.

My friend was in a coma, left in a vegetative state, and while his poor family grappled with the painstaking decision of whether to keep their son and brother on life support, they also asked that we not talk about what he and they were going through. This was their private and hopefully dignified moment.

After hearing this, I showed up late for practice the next day. I didn't say why, but somehow the media got wind of the accident, and word started to go around campus, word that, thanks to social media, turned ugly. One woman, for some reason, chose to take the accident and use it to attack me. Her posts were all about how I, as someone in the public eye, someone playing on the college football team, should be there for my friend. She stated that I hadn't done anything, or said anything, and portrayed me as the villain.

Compared to what my friend and his family were going through, her words, of course, didn't matter, but this opened my eyes to how people can simply say what they like, to a lot of people, and those words stick. She didn't care about

"YOU PLAYED WELL TODAY, SON"

what she said, or the facts around it. She didn't care about my friend, and she certainly didn't care about the truth.

She obviously hadn't said anything directly to me, because if she had, she would have discovered that my roommate's family asked us to keep our silence. Instead, thanks to the platform this lady had been given, the incident became ugly. That's when I first began to realize that social media could be a bad thing, and I soon deleted all my accounts.

In 2015, at my second Super Bowl with the Seahawks, the occasion was ruined by more than the fact that we lost to the Patriots. This time, my parents made it to the game, as did my two sisters. So, when a woman began to post on social media and then went to gossip blogs, stating that she was in town with me, and that I had paid for her to be there – that was an interesting situation.

Of course, I had a girlfriend at the time, my high school sweetheart, the one who had moved to Seattle with me. I had my mom and my sisters there, reading this stranger's posts. My mom had brought me up to be respectful to women, she knew I had a girlfriend, and she also always taught my sisters to deal only with good men. And there I was, trying to focus on the big game while all this talk was going on about me, but I found myself having to explain to my girlfriend that this other girl wasn't telling the truth. I did not look like a good guy.

People like this girl (I knew her, and she admitted that she just wanted to get my attention) have been around for so long, using newspapers to spread lies, but social media is so much more powerful, so much more immediate, and those lies reach far more people. It has its benefits, but I feel that too many people on these sites care little for their actions, and have no idea how much idle thoughts can hurt people and cause mental health issues. Yes, even for football players whose days are spent being hit by men weighing 300 pounds.

On top of social media, there was the constant quest for perfection, the blow of even the slightest failure or smallest mistake. The work you put in, that was never enough. You could strive all week, give it your all at practice, and come game day, mistakes would be made (that's sports), and you would be portrayed as nothing more than a chump. Opinions swirled around football players' lives. It was as if we weren't human, as if we were characters in a video game, and when the fourth quarter ended, it was simply "game over". Well, it wasn't.

Players listened to those opinions, all the talk that didn't allow for human error. "Everyone makes mistakes"? Not in pro football. People talked – the game belongs to the people who watch it, I understood that – but without knowing anyone involved, assumptions were made. The hurtful remarks echoed, and the person beneath the helmet got ignored. However hard we worked, it would be a guy who'd never even picked up a football in his life, sitting on his couch, typing his thoughts on social media who shaped conversations.

For all the physical attributes, all the weights lifted, the speeds achieved, the technical abilities, if a player's mental strength wavered, or if he was suffering quietly, that man on his couch with his cellphone could be the cherry on top of a very stressful cake.

There were levels to it. I understood that I, like so many pros, was not Tom Brady. Brady would have had his own set of pressures. Keeping healthy being one, knowing that with one bad injury, it could all be over. The constant attention, the need to be perfect, the expectation of success. All of that would take its toll and have to be dealt with.

Being at his level would have brought stresses that differed from those that I and so many others experienced. This is not about comparisons, but plenty of things the average player went through took place out of the spotlight.

Take Doomsday. That is what players call Tuesdays in the NFL. It should be a good day, the NFL's mandatory rest day. However, while we took the time to recover from the weekend's exploits, this wasn't a day for relaxation. We all knew what was going on. Every Tuesday, from around 10am to noon, about 15 to 20 guys would be trying out for a place on our teams, and if any of them were successful, they would get a place on the team – and one of us already on the roster would be out.

They came from everywhere. Flown in. We called them "off the street," and they consisted of guys who were out of contract, free agents, guys who weren't drafted but were still trying to make their dream come true. And if it did, *my* dream could have been over. It was that simple.

I might have played well on the Sunday, but come Tuesday afternoon, because a guy "off the street" had done well in my position, I might have been cut. It happened every week, all around the country. Doomsday. You were powerless. You just waited and hoped that, come Wednesday morning when you were back in for practice, you didn't get the news. "Sorry BJ, not this week."

Not only was there the broken ambition, but financially, the risk was huge. Yes, you had a contract, but should you be cut from the team, your finances were severely affected, so being part of the playing roster was vital. It got into your head. Tuesdays came around quickly, and there was always that worry. *Would it be me this week?*

Being in the NFL was hard on my mental health at the best of times, and I'm sure it still is for those in the league now. Working to be in the perfect physical shape required to be successful, striving to be the best teammate you can be, hoping that you are the perfect grandson, son and brother, despite living on the other side of the country. You want to be the perfect man, to be appreciated by your coaches and teammates, but the reality is, thanks largely to those Tuesdays, you are never really settled.

You live in a hotel, and the novelty quickly wears off. You rent a new apartment, but there is a nagging question at the back of your mind: *How long will I be here?* When I was playing, those Tuesdays became a sole focus. It should have been Sunday. Game day. All my thoughts should have been on that, being the best I could be, but instead it was Doomsday. Survive, pick up my check on Friday. Be involved and impress on the weekend, and move on to the next week. And so on. So many of us were stuck in a loop that could take its toll on the mind.

Let me reiterate: I loved being a pro football player, and being in the NFL, for me, was the ultimate dream. It is, however, important to highlight that from the moment you are drafted, things change, and some of it is hard. As soon

"YOU PLAYED WELL TODAY, SON"

as I took that call from the 49ers, in my parents' bathroom, I went from being BJ Daniels to NFL player BJ Daniels. It was inevitable.

The pride in my achievement and the happiness that was generated were both there, of course – but simmering away, under the surface, expectations crept in, expectations that affected people around me. BJ Daniels was an NFL football player, and he was also an immediate millionaire.

I could sense it. People looked at me, saw me differently. That was that. I'd made it. The mountain had been scaled. Everything was set. I had no more worries, and I could help them. No questions asked. People I didn't even know thought this way.

In my community, it became very apparent that as soon as I was drafted, I was seen differently. Among people, I had been "Brother". Often, my elders would see me as "Little Brother". Not anymore. Suddenly I was "Big Bro". Men older than me were calling me "Big Bro" because suddenly, in their minds, I was on a pedestal.

How am I your Big Bro? I'd think to myself. I wasn't anything to them before the draft, but now, because of my potential financial gains, I was a person who was respected, not for the hard work I had put in to get where I wanted to be, but for what I might have provided them. I also knew that when my pro career eventually ended, I wouldn't be anything to them then. I found it embarrassing and kind of sad. I wanted them to respect me for being me, not for what I might have given them or how I made them look.

Those early days as a pro football player were an eye-opener. The happiness I felt from making it definitely ran alongside a sometimes overpowering sense that I had been thrown into the lion's den without any weapons.

Moving to San Francisco, and then shortly after that to Seattle, all I wanted to do was make the team. But, and this is the same for so many drafted players, I was miles from home, and suddenly, I had agents all over me, I had a financial advisor (and I was figuring out if I could trust her advice), I had real estate agents chasing me, and I was far from financially literate, which I couldn't change right away, with practice and the start of the season taking up all my time.

It became consuming for me, and I can see that many young players still struggle. Their friends and family might be taking what they can from them or they, like me, will have a relationship that is hard to maintain due to both the change in circumstances and the new distance between them. It's a whirlwind, and with new teammates who they might not consider friends yet, it can be a time of intense learning that rookies have to take on alone. There's a three-month window in the early part of the year, post-season and pre-spring practice, and that is the time for players to get their affairs in order. Or learn how to. Welcome to the NFL, welcome to the team, but you have to figure out what it means to have money all by yourself.

For some players, it is too much. Some have a lot going on in their personal lives. They may have gambling issues, they may have the mother(s) of their child(ren) wanting things from them, they may have debts, or they may have already spent their first paychecks with reckless abandon, buying the nicest car on the lot before they have even made the team. Then, Doomsday comes, they're cut, and things begin to spiral. Their children's mothers are still on the phone, those debts are still hanging over them. There isn't much support or advice, and in the most extreme cases, young men give up or even take their own lives.

Suicide among football players is a huge concern, and a phenomenon that must be addressed. The 21st century has seen a notable rise in such cases, and while each man's story is unique, we should think about how the pressures of life surrounding the game – alongside the financial struggles I have mentioned, which increase when we take failed business ventures, divorce, family medical bills and (often forced) retirement into account – affect NFL players.

I never had thoughts about taking my own life, but I can totally empathize with the feelings of despair and emptiness that have led many of my peers to do so. I think back to my days starting out, and then moving around the country, trying to cement a place on a team, cement a place in the game.

I was so often alone, trying to make my relationship work, but without an apartment, and with the weekly Doomsday fight to stay on the team, I didn't move my girlfriend out to the West Coast immediately. Later, when I left Seattle (the only place in my career that gave me a sense of stability), I was in and out of hotel rooms, living out of a suitcase.

Even on the occasions when my girlfriend did come and live with me, there was a sense of distance between us, and because the career I wanted was so all-consuming, both my mental health and my behavior suffered. Suddenly, I couldn't rest, I couldn't relax. There was so much I was trying to achieve, nothing felt permanent – when all I craved was security – and I had no peace.

I would go to practice, give my all, and then rather than go home to be with my girlfriend or to just chill there and be with my thoughts, I would go out. Every day. To the nearest restaurant or bar, barbershop or the mall. I needed to be around other people, start conversations with bar staff, waiters, barbers or even strangers. I was looking for white noise, a distraction to take me away from my own thoughts.

That was a dangerous mental space to be in. I was far from settled, and that need to drown out the tension building within me could have spiraled and taken me to dark places: alcohol or drug dependency, other women, gambling. And all those could have been gateways to even darker places.

Looking back, I was lonely. And I felt that way when I was in the game, consumed by it, working with hundreds of people every day. Retiring and dropping out of the pro game is another challenge, but one that brings similar feelings of loneliness and self-doubt.

When my pro career ended, I found myself in a period of severe anxiety. The dream was over. I'd done everything I could to make it, but after I retired, there were feelings of failure, self-loathing and embarrassment. I stayed in Atlanta for a year, then moved back to Florida, and everyone said the right things, patted me on the back for a job well done. I was lauded for the efforts I'd made and the things I'd achieved. "There goes BJ Daniels. He won a Super Bowl ring, you know!"

"YOU PLAYED WELL TODAY, SON"

It was all very nice on the surface, but deep down, those words were boiling my blood. That Super Bowl ring meant less and less, the more I accepted that it was over. It wasn't even that I had to think hard about what I would do with my life; I just felt a very real anger that my time had come to an end. Anger with the system, anger with myself, anger with those voices trying to console me with what I felt were empty words.

The weekend would come around, and I couldn't stand to watch football. I wouldn't go near it, and I didn't care. I couldn't pick up the ball that, for nearly 30 years, I'd loved having in my hands. I now hated it. The thought of throwing it repulsed me. That ball symbolized a broken dream, reminded me of all the obstacles that eventually were too high to climb. My mind was broken. I refused to lift weights, I turned my back on playing pick-up basketball with friends. All these things that had always put a smile on my face, I shunned them, and with that, my personality changed. The smile went.

It's a common theme. An athlete retires, and a piece of them retires too. In some cases, that loss leads to extreme measures. As I said before, suicide among retired football players is also a serious issue. These are (still) young men, often in their late 20s, who were plucked from college, where their entire lives were organized for them, and then dropped into professional football and all the pressures that come with it, paid well, given little advice of how to manage that salary, and were often living their lives in a very insecure environment. Then, without any acknowledgment or advice, they are simply given a wave and told to get on with their lives.

Academic reports have suggested that mental health treatment given to retired professional athletes would help in so many cases that tragically lead to people taking their own lives. One case, that of Phillip Adams, was especially disturbing.

I knew Phillip. He was a teammate at the Seahawks. A sweet guy, fun, always smiling and working hard. But in 2021, I received a shocking text message from another one of my former teammates. Phillip had shot and killed six people: his therapist, his therapist's wife, two of their grandchildren, and two air-conditioning technicians working outside of the therapist's home. The next day, in a standoff with the police, Phillip took his own life.

I just couldn't believe it. Working with and getting to know Phillip, there was no sign of malice, nothing violent about him whatsoever. But when he retired from the game, the people around him said that he changed, his personality became more and more closed off, until something cracked, something that none of us can comprehend.

There was talk, of course. Some experts cited chronic traumatic encephalopathy (CTE), a neurodegenerative disease of the brain that occurs as a result of repeated head trauma, an issue linked to pro football, for obvious reasons. What hit me hard was hearing about Phillip's moods when he finished.

We had a lot in common. Like me, Phillip was drafted in the seventh round and moved from South Carolina to San Francisco. He moved from team to team, having a successful career (the average is three seasons; he played six), but he suffered a horrible ankle injury, and with younger, healthier guys available, he soon found that the phone calls from teams wanting to use his talents stopped coming in.

In 2016, the Indianapolis Colts did make a call, asking him to come and participate in a practice day. I'm not sure how many of these days he had been to, but I am more than aware of what it was like to travel, check into hotel after hotel, and feel all hope dwindling. Phillip got the airport, but he missed his plane. It was on that day that his former agent noticed a shift. "He made it to the Charlotte airport, but the flight had left already," his agent told *The New York Times*. "I could tell his head was not in it. He'd given up on it."[2]

From there, it is said that he experienced financial troubles. "His mental health degraded fast and terribly bad," his sister told *USA Today*. "There was unusual behavior."[3] From there, he saw a therapist, but when he stopped taking the medication he had been on, it seems that he cracked.

This remains an extreme and incredibly tragic case, one with many layers, but one that must have the NFL asking itself how it can help young men coming out of the league. That help must come in the form of medical attention and checks for conditions such as CTE, as well as support for the mental strain that comes with leaving their game.

Cases such as Phillip Adams's leave our communities with only heartbreak and questions. Could we have done more? Should we have seen the signs? Were we there for those involved? The truth is, depression doesn't have an outward sign we can look for. There are no physical traits, and with young men, there is often no call for help.

In my time as a player, if I was hanging out with, say, Marshawn Lynch, and there was something going on in one of our lives, something that was hurting our mental health, chances are, neither of us would bring it up. We would hang out, talk about the coaches, the upcoming game, the last game, girls, maybe a car we'd seen, but the big stuff, the heavy stuff that was taking its toll on us, that stayed locked away. We might have been friends, we were very close, but that was a door that we kept locked.

Today, I work with college students, athletes, young men and women with dreams and lives ahead of them, but many of them will carry doubts and feel burdened by dark thoughts. Now, they won't have a neon sign above them telling me that they are going through hell, but through my experiences, I have learned that interacting with people leads to conversation, and conversations can lighten a person's load.

Talking to people, it can make all the difference. As I said before, basketball legend Charles Barkley is a good friend of my uncle, Paul. They played at Auburn together. Charles has always told a story that stayed with me.

Charles and Paul were out one night at a party. By now, Charles was a big deal, a young man who was clearly going to the top of the NBA. But there was a guy at the party who wanted to make it clear he doubted this. He kept poking at Charles, trying to get a reaction out of him, all night long. This guy was saying that Charles was too fat, that his game wasn't good, that he was not nearly as talented as people were saying. Eventually, Charles got tired of him, so he picked him up and threw him out of the window.

Outside, the guy stood up, dusted himself off, put his hands in the air and shouted, "Yeah! Charles Barkley just touched me and threw me out of a window!" For Charles, it was an eye-opening moment, one that he took with him into his incredible career. Charles realized that if doing something as negative and dramatic as hurling this guy out of the window could have a positive effect, imagine what he could do for people by being nice.

My uncle has told me that, from that night on, he noticed how Charles would always engage with people who approached him. I have seen it too. Charles will be swamped by people wanting a piece of this time, and he is always polite, asking questions about their lives, making them laugh, and you can see that his actions have an uplifting effect on those around him. As for the guy who was thrown out of that window, I'm sure he's still milking that story.

I, of course, have never gotten as much attention as Charles gets, but I have tried to learn from people like him, so now, when I talk to students or anyone else, for that matter, I make sure that I'm engaged. Whatever is being said, positive or negative, I focus on the person talking. I encourage their thoughts, pay them a compliment, ask questions. Specifically, I ask them two things: Tell me one thing that's good in your life today, and tell me one thing that is bad. Ask someone those two things, and they will open up like a book. Show an interest in people, hear their stories, and you could make a difference. You never know what a person is going through – being in that moment with them, you will bring some light into their lives.

Even with this mindset, I can still have bad days. Maybe work gets on my nerves, or I'm frustrated because I feel unmotivated. Maybe people in the gym annoyed me, guys at basketball tried to provoke me, press my buttons. So, I go home in a terrible mood.

I'll walk in the house, still carrying all the negativity of the day, ready to let it define my evening. But then, I'll call my dad, hear about his day and talk about mine, and all that stuff on my shoulders drops. By talking to someone, hearing their good news, things within us can shift.

I guess it's all about communication. With those we know and love, but also with those we don't. In pro football, possibly the most macho environment there is, communication is key on the field, but when it comes to matters of the mind and heart, it isn't always there, so the dark clouds can gather.

Today, the notion of men talking about their problems is no longer greeted with raised eyebrows. Football might still be slightly behind, but we now appreciate that, beneath the pads and under the helmet, there is just a guy, and he might be having a hard time. I hope he knows that he is not alone.

9

SLEEPLESS IN SEATTLE

DEALING WITH FRUSTRATION AND UNCERTAINTY

Cry baby – that's what they used to call me. Through my elementary school years, and if I'm being perfectly honest, into middle school, I had that nickname. If my team was losing, then the tears would be running. It didn't matter if it was football, basketball, baseball or even the odd soccer game I played when I was very young – at the end of the game, if my team had lost, my mom and dad were going to have to deal with a very upset child.

It still happens today. Okay, I may not need tissues or a shoulder to cry on anymore, but if I go to the local community center to play some pick-up basketball, yes, I am going for some exercise, yes, I enjoy the cardio workout it gives me, but trust me, I am going there to win the game. When that doesn't happen, I don't like it. I don't like it at all.

But on the first night of February in 2015, in Glendale, Arizona, at the University of Phoenix stadium, I stood in a locker room with a big group of guys – players, coaches, staff – and saw a clear demonstration of what real frustration is, what it looks like and sounds like.

CRASH, a bench collided with the lockers. *BANG*, a chair broke into pieces after being thrown at a wall. Players were unloading on the coaches, screaming in their faces.

I stood there, unable to take in what had just happened. Emotions were running wild. Anger, frustration, despair, tears, even laughter at those unable to comprehend a defeat in such circumstances. The Seahawks had come so close to winning back-to-back Super Bowls, but right at the end, with just a couple of yards between us and our dreams, it all went wrong.

In sporting terms, it was the night that the New England Patriots beat the Seattle Seahawks to win Super Bowl XLIX in dramatic fashion. The night that Tom Brady won the fourth of his eventual seven rings, the night the world witnessed arguably the most exciting Super Bowl in history. For the Seahawks, though, for those on the squad who had come together and achieved so much, it was a night that saw something in the team die, something that had made the team so, so special.

***

The 2014–15 season had started well. The team and the city were still on a high. We were the first Seahawks team to win the Super Bowl, and as we discovered when we reunited there in 2023, that is something that will remain ingrained in the fabric of the city. People's hearts are filled by that level of success, and we were able to really enjoy the achievement.

To win, to be the best in the country, to do something that huge, you could see what it meant to the city. The thing about Seattle and its people is that they feel a little ignored. They are on the West Coast, but they are not in California, which seems to get all of the attention. Meanwhile, people hear "Seattle" and only think of the rain, Amazon's headquarters, or maybe the TV show *Frasier*. They may also mention the suicide rates there, which once were the highest in the country, but it's typically nothing positive. They don't talk about how beautiful the city and its surrounding areas are, especially in the spring, or the jaw-dropping coastline, mountains and forests.

For a long time, they didn't really mention the football team either. But now they did, and they did so a lot. The whole country was watching, and for the locals, that was something to celebrate, to be able to stand up above everyone else and say we were the best.

It was a great feeling, so starting the 2014–15 season, all of us – players, coaches, staff and the locals – were desperate to feel that glory again. Going into the season, a couple of players had moved on, but we kept our core mentality from the year before. There was a real hunger, a sense that we could go again and achieve what so few teams had by winning the big one back-to-back. Why not? We had the team, we had the coach, we had the people firmly behind us, and we had each other.

We weren't winning quite as ruthlessly as we had the previous year, but still finished the regular season 12–4, before beating the Carolina Panthers in the divisional playoffs, and then facing the Green Bay Packers in the NFC Championship, which took place in Seattle.

The game proved to be a learning curve. We were down 16–0, and frankly, we were getting our butts kicked. It was a humbling game, one that forced us to refocus and realize that if we didn't play hard, our hardest, then we would get beat. The team had to find our grit and determination to overcome being down 19–7 with just five minutes to go. Not many other teams could have turned it around, force the game into overtime and eventually win 28–22. But we did.

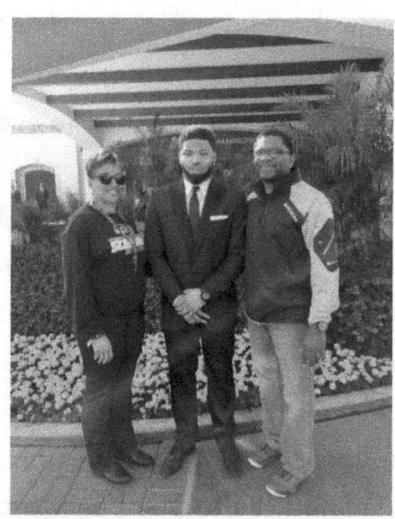

My parents and me before Super Bowl XLIX, 2015

So, we headed to another Super Bowl, this time in Arizona, for a final showdown against the New England Patriots, and they were no joke. If the Denver Broncos, with Peyton Manning at the helm, had the odds in their favor the year before, then the Patriots, and their then three-time Super Bowl-winning quarterback, Tom Brady, were once again on another level.

I was back-up quarterback that night, but there was also a chance I could play wide receiver, and as a team, we knew that we would have to draw on all our inner strengths if we were going to win. And that's exactly how it went. Two great teams, going toe to toe, extreme talent on both sides, no one giving an inch, but then, at the end, that's what it came down to: inches.

Everyone who watches football knows what happened at the end, the play that was called, the Russell Wilson throw just yards from the end zone that was intercepted by a rookie free agent named Malcolm Butler. With just seconds left, the world turned upside down, and the Patriots took the title, 28–24.

"I cannot believe the call," was the commentator's immediate reaction. For days, newspaper columns, online articles and social media pages were filled with debate about who was to blame. Why wasn't the ball just handed off to Marshawn Lynch? He was a 240-pound running back with the nickname "Beast Mode" – a grown man that could run through a wall – and we just needed a yard to win. Who made the call? How did Pete Carroll allow for such an error?

Roughly 114 million people were watching that night, so there were always going to be opinions, and at the heart of it was, of course, my fellow quarterback, Russell Wilson. What those many voices didn't take into consideration was that the play was by no means called or carried out by mistake or without thought.

Russell threw the ball, but he certainly didn't call the play, and in defense of whoever did, that was a play that we'd successfully done a hundred times. It wasn't new – we had done it in practice, we had done it in games – but then, there, on that occasion, in the most dramatic setting possible, with all eyes on us, it went wrong, and the world was immediately judging us all. It's a tough game.

What was also hard was the night out after such a devastating loss. A year earlier, I had witnessed the faces of the Broncos players out in New York watching us celebrate our win. We were now in their shoes, asked to be present at a party with the devastation of what had just happened, basically to drown our sorrows.

It wouldn't be easy, especially after the aggression that had been shown in our locker room after the game. The Seahawks arranged for a party in the hotel after the game. There was food and an open bar, and the organization wanted us to celebrate a "successful season," but even with Snoop Dogg there performing for us, as cool as that always was, how could we celebrate anything?

We had come together in the spring, we had worked hard through the preseason, played every game with our focus on going all the way. And then we fell short by a yard. How could we celebrate? The season was over.

***

Looking back, after that night, it wasn't just the season that had ended – the special energy between the team did, too. To lose the way we did and face so much negativity for a single play – something changed, something left us, a trust was broken. The locker room arguments that saw some players cussing out coaches and vice versa, they sped up the process. Players were wondering who called the play. There were whispers about the offensive coach, about whether Russell was up to the job. Could he have changed the play, or was he looking for the glory of a winning touchdown pass? It was all a mess. It broke us apart.

It got to the point where it became toxic and, suddenly, with our trust gone, the glue that kept us together disappeared too. That night in Arizona, I think the world witnessed the death of a football team. We started as a team of young players, many of us told "no" by other teams, all of us driven by the glory of the game and wanting to lift each other up. And then, all of a sudden, there were cracks. Some guys were just not fully there after that loss. Players were looking forward, wondering where else they could play, thinking about the financial gains they could make if they moved on. Everything had changed.

In many ways, I had, too. It had been a mind-altering year at the Seahawks. The victories, the success, the sense of belonging in the NFL that I gained in Seattle, with hindsight, I can say now that a lot of it went to my head.

My girlfriend and I, while living together and continuing to make our relationship work, were never on firm ground, and with my success in football, I became less tolerant. If things didn't go my way with her, my attitude turned colder, more arrogant. *Okay, if you don't like things this way, I'll find someone who does* was a constant thought.

I think it was the access that success had afforded me that went to my head. Success had given me the opportunity to see so much, to meet so many people. Suddenly I was friends with Drake, hanging out with him, traveling to Vegas to celebrate our shared birthday. I was experiencing real celebrity. I was walking into rooms and getting a lot of attention. With it, my patience became thinner, and that arrogance I mentioned started to creep in.

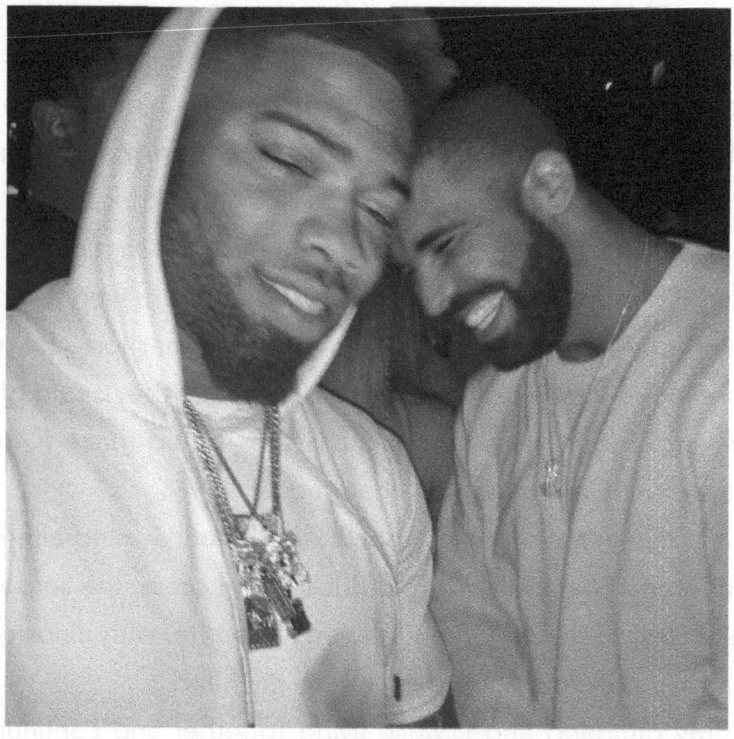

Me and Drake

If I am honest with myself, having reached the NFL, being involved in those huge games, that was all very special, but I hadn't become the man I truly wanted to be. I could have used the platform that my hard work had given me for so much more. I didn't take the time to invest in myself, to set myself up for the future.

Instead, I was consumed with the environment I was in, and the access I had to what I thought were the finer things. Being young, I thought it would all last forever; there was no time in my mind to consider life after football. Relationships or thoughts about the future, they didn't matter. I refused to share anything with football – I chose the sport over everything. I didn't invest in a business or myself. My relationship and even friendships took a back seat. I was only living for the moment. I was young, I was a pro football player with a Super Bowl ring, and I was rolling with it.

Eventually, as that feel-good vibe felt by the team started to disappear, so did my own happiness. The first year was great. I learned so much. But now, in my second year with the Seahawks, I started to come to work feeling paranoid. Every Tuesday, that Doomsday feeling kicked in.

Were they looking at other players to replace me? Did I have the coach's trust and admiration? It had become hard to tell, but I began to lose confidence in my place in Coach Carroll's heart. Right before the 2015–16 season, they invited three other quarterbacks to training camp. That set the tone. With Russell and I already there, the quarterback room started to get busy, so practice offered me much fewer chances to shine.

The frustrations and that paranoia began to set in, and that's when I started to make changes. Play me anywhere. If quarterback was so full, if they felt the need to look at three others, then why not try me somewhere else? The decision went against my firm self-belief that I was a quarterback, but that had been replaced by a deep desire to play, and I was now going to do whatever it took to get on the field.

I remained a back-up QB, but I spread myself thin. Wide receiver, okay, running back, yes, special teams, punt returner, I said yes to everything, and for a while it worked. I was getting game time; every week I had the opportunity to get out there.

Wide receiver was the main position I was told to play. That meant I had to change everything. I dedicated the whole off-season in 2015 to working on and essentially changing my physique. Playing at wide receiver, there is so much more strain on your whole body. You're running more, sprinting, twisting, stopping, starting. I had done it a bit over the years, but now I was preparing to do it consistently, and that meant changing my body and my mentality.

My weight had to change, as did my physicality, my diet and my routine. Here I was again, like in high school and college, having to prove my ability. It crossed my mind that I thought I was done with all that, but my desire to play every week fueled my work.

Then, we got to summer training camp, and I was up against 15 other wide receivers, and we all knew they would only take 8 of us into the season. What hit me was that I was competing against guys who had played in that position for their entire athletic careers. Not only that, but I was learning the role against world-class defensive players ("The Legion of Boom"). But I had to try it – and I gave it my all.

Much of my work, away from the weight room, was on the technique and what it meant to play at wide receiver. Compared to many, I wasn't the fastest, so I concentrated on how to get open. Movement, quick thinking and agility.

I worked hard – very hard. I kept my head down, learned, didn't complain, but there was, for the first time in Seattle, a sense of frustration and the feeling that I was no longer loved by the staff. I had done all that was asked as back-up QB, but now it felt that Coach Carroll, a man I had grown so fond of, was telling me that I wasn't good enough. From Pete, that hurt.

But I couldn't show that hurt; I just had to keep going, do what I could. Those were my thoughts, and today, I regret them. I should have stood my ground, been the young man I was in high school and when being recruited by colleges. *I am a quarterback.*

What was hard was that they brought in a new quarterback for preseason practice, and I could see, early on, that he was not better than me. That was not me being conceited. How did I know that? Because I was playing receiver, and he was throwing to me. I watched him play, caught his passes, and I knew I was better than him. In the end, I made the team, and he didn't. That's crazy.

For the first three preseason games, I played receiver and did okay. Then, in the fourth, one of our quarterbacks got hurt, and they put me in. Now, I had not taken a snap or worked on any plays for months, but there I was. Sneakily, I had thrown some passes in practice. I would receive a pass, sprint 40 or 50 yards for conditioning, but instead of strolling back and simply giving the ball back to the ball boy, I would throw it all the way back. I wanted to make sure, that even if I was having to change myself, I still had my range.

In that preseason game against the Oakland Raiders, I came in at quarterback and threw a touchdown pass. It was a surreal moment, one that had my mind in overdrive, yearning to be in that position. But it also showed my teammates that I was a team player, that I could work hard and be productive wherever I was asked to play. I sensed the respect I'd earned, and while the coaches had become slightly standoffish with me, to see that approval from my peers meant so much.

I think the coaches started to see me as the utility guy, and any football player can tell you that is never good. If you can play in various positions, while you're invaluable to the team, you also become a possible afterthought. "There's a problem? BJ will go there." And if you won't, well, they'll find someone younger, cheaper and more willing to step in. When I was in the NFL, there was joke among players that we needed to do whatever it took to be on that field, or we'd end up working at Walmart. That was what was on my mind, and while I have come to regret my decision to switch positions, being young and desperate to play, I did all I could do.

But all I could do would too often not be enough. I would be on the active 53-man roster, I'd play in the games, and then on Doomsday, I would get cut and put on the practice squad. The next week, the Seahawks would bring me back. It started to feel like they were playing with my emotions because getting cut on a Tuesday meant I couldn't play in the game on Sunday. I didn't know if I was leaving or staying.

My head was spinning. I would play, do well, show off all the new skills I'd learned: playing receiver, playing on special teams, returning punts, learning to tackle, plucking balls out of the sky from 100 feet – trust me, a football looks like a dot when it's falling from that height. Then the following week, I would be dressed, ready, and I wouldn't play. I was cut twice and brought back, and then one morning it happened again: The grim reaper approached me.

"Are we really going to do this again?" I asked.

"Don't shoot the messenger," was his reply.

We walked up to the office of the general manager, John Schneider, and I was mad. Visibly so. Schneider was sitting in his chair, and he could tell that I was not happy. How could I be? I knew what he was about to say. I got cut again.

"It's a numbers thing, BJ," he told me.

I'd heard it before.

"We can only keep a certain number of people, and as much as we'd love to have you on the team, we have to put you back on the practice squad."

Not only did they take away my spot on the team, but they took a big chunk of my salary. Again.

"Ok, John," I said. "I get that it's a numbers game, but how come I am always the one in the count?"

John didn't answer. He had no answers. I was cut again. Sorry, and see you later. I turned to leave, wondering if there *would be* a later. So, before I left, I looked back at him and simply said, "John, how would you feel if it was your son?" Again, there was no answer.

That week, back on a waiver, my mind was set on leaving. I still had the same agent who was with me during the draft. To be honest, I was still learning the industry and leaned too much on him. I'd listen to the guys in the locker room, learning from them about the league and realizing that I had to be more aggressive with matters regarding my own future.

I wanted to be marketed by my agent in the right way. I didn't want him to just handle my career – I wanted to be involved, but that took experience. The thing about becoming an NFL player is that it kind of happens overnight. You get drafted, and then what? Well, the NFL then invites you to their Hall of Fame offices in Canton, Ohio.

There, you join every drafted rookie, and for three days they talk at you. We were told about girls, the pitfalls of nightclubs, agents and some financial issues. Then, after three days, they said goodbye, and off we went to our new teams' cities. Three days of talks? To me, that was nowhere near enough – it seemed like they were just checking a box.

Off we all went to New York, Miami, San Francisco, Chicago. These big cities awaited us, and we – armed with a few days' worth of vague information and advice – headed off to live our adult lives. I found it weird then, and it still baffles me now. More needs to be done to teach these young men about their money and an industry that will, when given the chance, chew them up and spit them out.

Without help from the NFL, I did most of my learning by listening to teammates. From them, I got some good ideas about how I wanted my career, my business, to be handled. I now, despite the amount of love and affection I had for the Seahawks, knew my worth, and the routes I wanted to take.

So, the day after exiting John Schneider's office and ending up back on the waiver, my agent was on the phone. He called to tell me that the Houston Texans wanted to take me, and should I agree, they'd want me at quarterback. I was immediately interested. If I went, they would give me the chance to compete as the starting quarterback. They were big and bold words, the ones that I wanted to hear for so long. I didn't need to think about it at all. This was a no-brainer. I was off to Texas.

Football, like so many sports, is a cutthroat and detached business when it comes to departures and goodbyes. If the Seahawks had based their success on that family-like connection, then that wasn't evident when I left. Just days later, my locker was cleaned out, my bags were packed, and I was on a flight to join another team.

I liked Houston immediately. I liked the Texans' staff and team and their warmth, so I threw myself into practice. Maybe a little too hard. It was now December 2015, and I had spent the entire season up to that point at wide receiver. Those throws I'd snuck in at practice with the Seahawks were a good start – I still had the distance – but the strength in my throwing arm had suffered. Going in cold and throwing at quarterback again, I tore a small muscle in my shoulder that meant I couldn't play at 100 percent. Any velocity I hoped to achieve with my throwing, and my career, was stalled.

Houston, and the head coach, Bill O'Brien, a hardcore guy, could use me for the athletic ability I had worked on in Seattle, though. I was played in the few games left of that season (we lost in the Wild Card playoffs) as a wildcat quarterback, running plays, going in at key moments. Was it my ideal role? Not at all – the injury was hugely frustrating. However, I was happy to be back at quarterback, I was wanted by my team, and I was on the field every week.

There was no paranoia, and Tuesdays were no longer Doomsdays because I felt like my spot on the team was secure. On top of that, Houston fans had noticed me as a hardworking player, who, having come from one of the best teams in the NFL, could and would improve their team's chances in the future.

The future? I had been very much living in the moment in Seattle, as a young football player in love with the moment and the limelight that came with it. But in Texas, my mind moved forward. This could be a place I had a future. The team liked me, I liked the team, the people welcomed me with Texan charm, and while my life and all my belongings were in my apartment a couple of thousand miles away in Seattle, I allowed myself to think about the long term.

I spent the offseason getting healthy, fixing my shoulder and preparing for a real shot at being an NFL starting quarterback. It was so exciting for me. I signed a two-year contract, a long time in the NFL, and counted down the days to spring camp. Desperate to get started, to be the player at the center of it all, the season couldn't come fast enough.

But then it didn't come at all. Bad news was never given elaborately in the NFL. There was no fanfare. It was just short, sharp and deadly. As it turned out, the Texans' owners and general manager had decided to go in another direction. That meant bringing in a new quarterback. That also meant cutting me.

As simple as that. But what about the contract? Owners and general managers have all the power, and that means they, unlike the player, can make and break contracts. It's one of the dark, gritty sides of the industry. That contract I signed, one that I thought signified some security, was nothing but paper and ink, and I couldn't do anything about it.

If you ask me today, I think there is something players can do about it, and it means coming together and saying, "Enough." The fact that players can be dropped so easily, that contracts can be torn up with no fear of financial payback, is simply not good enough, and action – whether it's the biggest names in football speaking out or teams going on strike – should be a priority in *all* players' minds.

The problem is there are not enough of them willing to put themselves out there and inspire real change. Things might be said here and there, complaints might be made, but those at the top get on with their lives and spend $300,000 on a new car, $60,000 on a night in the strip club, thousands on an outfit they will wear once just for the Instagram picture they'll post for their millions of followers.

Those are the top guys. Those are the guys whose voices will count. Not enough of them are willing to suggest going on strike, saying they simply won't play until these contract situations are changed. The guys earning the lowest salaries in the NFL can't strike alone, and they need their salaries to take care of their families and put food on the table. If the guys who are on $200 million contracts take a stand, then, yes, suddenly you might have the world's attention. The situation needs help from the people at the top. That's how the future generation of players will be helped. These guys who need support aren't the superstars, but I can tell you this: There would be no NFL without them.

Pro football is a tough business. Hundreds of millions of television screens show the games each week, but viewers won't always notice how quickly players come and go. But remember, these are real people – they are not statistics, they are not robots. They are young men, and many of them are working beyond hard to make their dreams come true.

For me, that dream was still there, even after I got cut from the Texans. I was on the road again, wondering what was around the corner, but as I pondered my next move, what I was sure about was my ability to make it. I remember feeling rejected, but having that fire inside me still burning. *Just put me in the game*, I'd think. *Just put me in the game and see me.*

The ability was there, that was how I had gotten as far as I had, but what I wanted to show consistently was my passion, mentality and desire. There was the speed, the mobility, the arm strength. There was also the fact that I could do everything normal quarterbacks could do, but I was also super mobile, and frankly, ahead of my time.

Today, Lamar Jackson, Patrick Mahomes, Baker Mayfield – they are all seen as mobile, dual-threat quarterbacks. I could have been like them. I just needed a chance.

The phone soon rang. Where would I be going next?

10

THE STRUGGLE TO SURVIVE

FIGHTING SELF-DOUBT TO STAY IN THE GAME

The clock is ticking. On the game of life, and maybe my football career. We're in the last preseason game before the 2016–17 season starts. I am wearing, yet again, a new uniform: this time, it's the Chicago Bears. We are facing the New England Patriots, who are winning by a touchdown. The clock is ticking. We're on the 50-yard line, and I'm at wide receiver. A last-second, desperate heave toward the end zone is all we have time for. Hail Mary.

By a hospital bed in Daytona Beach, Florida, my family is all gathered. My beloved grandmother, Ewlillie, has cancer, an illness that has taken control of her body, so much so that many of my relatives have made the journey to be with her. They have a television in her room, so the game is on, and as always, my grandma is focused on me, excited to see me doing what I love, no matter what's happening to her or the insignificance of who wins a preseason game.

My family is there, and I am in uniform, hundreds of miles away. My mind is on my grandmother, but my short-term focus is on the play at hand. The quarterback takes the snap and drops back. I'm off. I run down the middle of the field, passing the linebackers. As I look back, I see I'm being chased by Patriots defenders, but I'm hoping for the chance to make the game-winning touchdown. Just as I reach the end zone, I notice the ball is in the air. I jump in the air with my arms outstretched. The football falls right into my hands as I tap my feet on the grass, just inside of the field of play. Touchdown.

In the hospital, my sister happened to be recording the scene, and she turned her camera on my grandmother's bed at that very moment as she started to wildly cheer. There she was, her body taken over by a cancer that wasn't going to go away, but her spirit couldn't be held down. In what was a hard time for the family and her, she found a reason to celebrate, as her grandson scored a touchdown. The whole game, I played with that vision in my mind: I wanted to score a touchdown for her, and I did it in the very last second of the game.

It was a game that meant nothing to either team, nothing more than a warm-up to something far, far bigger. But there, in that hospital room, and to me miles away thinking of them all, it meant the world. The next day, the Chicago Bears cut me from the season's playing roster. By then, I had spoken to my family and been told about the joy that touchdown had brought my grandmother. The decision by the Bears to let me go might have, at another time in my life, made me angry or frustrated. Instead, I left grateful for the opportunity they had given me. My mind and heart were with my family. I had peace.

***

I needed it. After being told I was not wanted by the Houston Texans, I had become troubled and uncertain. Sure, I had that firm belief in my ability as a football player – that had not gone away – but that assurance not being matched by another team, another general manager, that was starting to erode my self-worth.

After those games with the Texans and signing a contract there, my girlfriend and I decided to give it another shot. She had been with me in Seattle but left, and with what I thought was a real chance at the NFL in Houston, we hoped, this time, football could help make it work.

She came out, we searched for a home, and we found one. Two bedrooms, a garage, wood floors – a real grown-up home where we could build a grown-up relationship. Everything I owned in Seattle was packed up and shipped to Houston, and as it was unpacked, I was standing there, thinking that perhaps this time, something might be built. A life.

And then, it happened. Houston told me the news: I was cut. When it happens, your mind spins with thoughts. Practically, there was the frustration that I wouldn't even get to show them how I could play, injury-free. I was also angry that, during the season, with a roster of 53 players, I was deemed good enough (with an injury) to play, and now in the preseason, with a roster of around 90 guys, they didn't think – even when I was healthy – that I was good enough.

So many thoughts, so many unanswered questions. My ego was dented, and the more dents I got, the more I started to fear fatal holes. I had been on one of the best squads, if not the best squad in the NFL with Seattle. I wanted to play, so I agreed to join, with all due respect, one of the more mediocre teams in the league. I did well under the circumstances, but even though they gave me that contract, they decided to try rookies and free agents ahead of me. It bothered me, not just from an egotistical perspective, but because I planned on making a life there. My girlfriend moved to be with me, and she was expecting security; my grandmother was diagnosed with cancer, and my paychecks were helping pay for that treatment; and I was paying for my sister's community college fees. I felt responsible to provide for them, not just because I loved my family, but because of their unwavering support throughout my life and especially my football career. But now, every road I went down seemed to be a dead end.

It was a time full of turmoil. After getting cut by the Texans, I drove to our house, to the home we were trying to build (already on a shaky foundation between us), walked in, looked her in the eye, and told her that I just lost my job. That was so hard. From a man's perspective and that sense of masculinity that is ingrained in us, to have to say that I could not provide or sustain our home was very troubling.

I knew I had to return to Tallahassee, and as much as I love my parents, I was very disheartened by that option. Looking back, I think this was the most difficult time in my football career, a time when outside influences started creeping into my mind.

I would look at my social media, see what always looked like ideal lives being led by other players who I believed were not as good as me, and things being said by people who did not know the work I was putting in. It was then that I decided to delete all my social media. I had almost 100,000 followers

THE STRUGGLE TO SURVIVE

on Instagram, but there was only negativity, and that was having an impact on me and my mood.

What slightly lifted my spirits was a call from the New York Giants in May 2016. They wanted me to come in for a tryout. *Okay – let's do this.* They had signed a quarterback to their roster, given him a contract, paid him some money, but – and this underlines the lack of stability in the NFL – they were more impressed by me, so they cut the other guy and signed me instead. I can't lie, it felt good to be on the other side of what I'd just experienced in Houston.

In New York, the city I had always loved, I picked up where I left off: studying the playbook, getting noticed in practice and learning from great players such as Eli Manning and Odell Beckham Jr. They later became good friends of mine, especially Odell, and because of these relationships, I allowed myself (yet again) to wonder if my future, which had been shrouded in mystery for so long, might be here.

For the Fourth of July, the Giants gave us a couple of weeks off, so I went back to Florida, and it was there that I received a call. Another call. The call. It seemed the Giants were signing someone else, and I wasn't to go back. I asked who it was, and when they told me it was Logan Thomas, it dawned on me that it was happening again. They had gone for the typically tall (6-foot-6), heavier guy, the guy who checked the boxes of what they thought a quarterback should be and look like.

I was devastated. For the first time ever, I started to think that football, for me, might be over. It was a traumatic thing to think, a traumatic thing to consider. I was back home, and while I was with people I love so much and who love me back, it was not where I wanted to be.

I had some money in my pocket, savings, but it felt scary to be home, like a sign that my dream was over. With every old face I saw, I sensed their thoughts: *Oh well, BJ, you gave it your best, but that's it, you're one of us now. You're just like the rest of us.* The thing was, I never wanted to be like the rest of them.

There are plenty of people who I went to school with, who do all of their living in Tallahassee. They go to school there, get married there, work there, die there. That is fine, of course, but I had different ideas, and to walk around and realize that people thought I was done, well, I didn't like it.

I'd had some fame and that brought jealousy from some people I used to know, a bad feeling that I had somehow got lucky or that I was privileged. I'd see girls who never looked at me when we were in school, but now, with the NFL attached to my name, they wanted to get to know me. On the other hand, I lost friendships with people who felt I'd abandoned them when I left town. Plenty of old friends were either in jail, on drugs or dependent on alcohol. So many different dynamics, and while I always knew Florida would eventually be my home again, I wasn't ready to begin that chapter of my life in Tallahassee.

That was when the Giants called me back. Logan Thomas had not been performing as well as they had hoped, and they wanted me to come back. I said no. That might sound crazy, given how much I wanted to get back into the game, but with all that happened, at that moment I felt this huge surge of self-worth. I was tired of being messed around.

Their call made me realize that I could absolutely be an asset in the game, but not at the risk to my own principles. Maybe it was because I was at home, and that environment reminded me of my struggles in school and with college recruitment. Those experiences showed me who I was – a short, Black quarterback who was more than capable in the position. I wouldn't compromise then, and I shouldn't compromise for the Giants. So, it was a "no" to New York, and a "let's get back to work" to my agent.

So, that's what we did. I packed my bags once again and headed out to the Detroit Lions, to the New England Patriots and then to the Green Bay Packers. After all these tryouts, it soon dawned on me that my interests might not be aligned with those of the people on *my* team.

At first, I had felt that there was a real relationship with my agent. I'd seen *Jerry Maguire* and laughed at the closeness achieved between the titular character, a sports agent played by Tom Cruise, and his client, Cuba Gooding Jr.'s Rod Tidwell. It was probably naïve of me, but I hoped for the same relationship. But, as the years passed, I grew to understand that, in reality, the famous phrase from that movie, "Show me the money!" works both ways, and my agent only got paid if I got paid. I understood it. He had to look after himself as well as me.

It was clear that he was going into rooms with general managers and doing everything that it took to get me on the team. I am grateful for that, but at the time, I wanted to be pushed as a quarterback. The feeling that I needed to be true to myself was as strong as ever. "BJ Daniels, that's who I represent" is how I imagined the conversation to begin. "Will you give him an opportunity? He is a very good player, a few injuries, but he is good, and he can play in multiple positions. He is your utility guy. Give him a shot?"

That's not what I wanted. As I arrived at these tryouts, I worked my hardest, but it was clear that I was being sold as something I wasn't. Yes, I could play various positions, but I wasn't a specialist at any of them. At the Packers, after they had me work out at wide receiver, I had enough. I went to the coaches and said, "Let me throw."

They looked at me like I was crazy. Like they didn't even know I could throw.

"What do you mean?" they asked.

"Let me show you…"

There they were, those words that I had used so often throughout my life. "Let me show you." They hung there as I took the ball and started to throw. I had a great session, the ball flying out of my hands, and while I did not get signed, I had seen the shock on their faces. That was the thing. I was walking into rooms and onto fields, and had no resemblance to the typical guy who'd play in my position. Look at Tom Brady, the stereotypical pro-style quarterback, the body shape, that height. And then there was me, 220 pounds, wide shoulders, and thick, long arms. But I was in great shape. I looked like a free safety or a running back.

I came home again, I got those same looks from the locals, and I felt those same uncomfortable feelings within me – that old NFL joke about working at Walmart was always on my mind. I had no idea where my next paycheck was coming from. My grandma Ewlillie was suffering from cancer, and it was getting worse. We needed to pay for doctors to simply tell us what was happening, and it was hard for all of us. This was a woman who meant so much to us.

My father's mom, she was always the spiritual leader on that side of the family, and she and I, from the moment I was born, had a deep connection. She was a rock, someone who, when I was low, I could call on, and she was always checking in on me. She was so special. As a young boy, my grandfather, her husband, would tease me all the time. "Hey, see that BJ," he'd say to everyone, "he's one sorry dude."

My grandma would always step in, even though it was a joke.

"Don't talk about my boy like that!" she'd say.

I *was* her boy, and now that she needed medical treatments that cost money, I knew I had to get back to work. Soon, I'd see that even more clearly.

***

It had been a month since I turned down the Giants when the Chicago Bears called. I was getting tired of traveling around the country, trying out for teams and not making the cut, but I was also feeling like this was my last shot. Plus, I needed to work, so I flew to the Windy City and stayed the night in a hotel before another tryout in the morning. The next day, as I was getting dressed and ready to go, my mom called, and I could immediately tell that something was wrong. She told me that my sister Laurel had cancer. Hodgkin's lymphoma.

I didn't know what it was, but a volt of shock ran through my body. I am a guy who hears terms like "cancer", and hears that someone is going to the hospital, and I immediately think that they aren't coming out. I stayed on the phone, listening to my mom's words, wanting to be in Florida, but knowing that I had a tryout that now meant the world.

The workout that followed was for Laurel. I was determined to make it the best one I ever had. These tryouts are about teams and coaches looking at your ability, but they are also about ensuring you're in perfect shape. If you impress, you are joining that squad the next day, and that means being ready immediately. They tried to run us into the ground, but that day, however hard they tried to finish us, I found more energy. If they were wondering if anyone would give up, that day, they saw that I wouldn't, and I made the team.

I returned to my hotel, and I sat on the bed, full of emotion, but I didn't have time to let it take over. The news about Laurel hadn't completely sunken in yet. I barely had time to process it because I had given my all at tryouts, and I had to dive into my new position on the Bears immediately – I already had a playbook to study before practice the next day. It also wasn't lost on me that I had done it again, and my NFL dream was still alive. Making the team also gave me the chance to work, get paid and help my family, a responsibility I felt now more than ever.

I called my sister and my mom, who, being a nurse, explained everything. She told us about Laurel's type of cancer, and that because it had been diagnosed relatively early, it could be managed with care, and things could be okay. The word "could" is never an easy one for me to trust, though, especially while we were all dealing with my grandmother's diagnosis, too. It was a tough time for the Daniels family.

Reassured by my mom's positivity and knowledge, I went to work in Chicago with the same enthusiasm I showed at tryouts. It was late summer, so I'd missed the initial training camp, and I was therefore way behind the other preseason roster guys. I knew that I had an uphill battle, a playbook to learn, but I was composed, drawing on my experience and knowledge of the game, taking on the challenge with a calmness that maybe I didn't have before.

And then there was that last preseason game I already told you about, my game-winning touchdown, and subsequently being cut. What a time. But I left Chicago with a feeling of peace. I was in my grandmother's heart at that moment, and that thought changed something in me, made me realize that all of this, everything I was trying to achieve, was for something so much bigger than just the glory of sports.

Everything had been about me. Be a quarterback, make a ton of money, be a starter, throw touchdowns, throw more touchdowns, break records, have a million followers on Instagram, hang out in Miami with beautiful people. Me, me, me, me, me.

I was always a good person, I think. My family would have ensured that. All of them were in service careers, but my path, those athletic dreams, had given me tunnel vision that pointed me toward my goals, but didn't allow me to see a bigger picture.

I realized that during my career, pieces of me had been left all over America, scattered by the experiences that I had. What I didn't realize was that I was taking pieces from each place, too, nuggets of information that I would use one day. All the times they tried to break me, all the cuts (literal and metaphorical), all the times I had been told "no", all the disappointments – it could be used to make me a better person, and one day, I could help others who were going through similar moments in life.

It was when I realized this that things started to change for me. That constant struggle to still make it, being cut or rejected – it hit different now. My beloved grandmother and my sister, maybe it was what was happening to them that brought perspective. We were all going through so much, but I suddenly became aware that there was more to life, that I had more to strive for than just football. Soon after, my grandmother passed.

It was so hard. I had lost people before – friends, teammates – and it was never easy. But with someone who I'd grown up with, who cared so much, who was able to always make me feel better like she had when I was just a little boy, it was heartbreaking. I think losing your first grandparent can be a first insight into grief. My grandma was the blood of my blood, and it hit so hard.

I remember the funeral. I was a pallbearer, and the weight of the occasion was something I'll never forget. My father spoke that day. He spoke beautifully about his beloved mom, and I remember looking up to him (I always have, and I always will look up to him) as he spoke at the service. I thought to myself, *How is he able to do this?* He was hurting so bad, but his words and his strength underlined to me the sheer power he has within him.

I thought I was strong. I lifted weights. I'd brushed off defensive linemen. I was an NFL player, but as I sat there, feeling both grief and pride in equal measure, I saw that it was my dad, this man who had guided me on my journey, who was the strong one. Tears began to roll down my cheeks, and as I helped to carry my grandma from the service, they rolled harder and harder. I didn't care. I didn't care what people saw or who they thought this athlete was *supposed* to be. That day, I witnessed real strength, and I realized that breaking down and showing emotion was nothing to be ashamed of.

***

With all that happened with my sister and grandmother, alongside a summer spent looking for a team, that change in me that I mentioned, allowed me to find as much focus as possible. My mind was relatively clear. What was important was obvious, and while I had two months without work, I continued to believe that football was my future.

I trained by myself, and I trained hard. I was in the gym, lifting weights and playing a lot of basketball, mainly because it's great cardio work and I hate running. (I can run, I am good at running, but I don't like it.) These workouts ensured I was in good shape when the call came that the Atlanta Falcons were interested in trying me out.

It was exciting news, made better by the fact that the head coach there was Dan Quinn, a great man who I had worked with closely at the Seahawks. Coach Quinn had been the defensive coordinator in Seattle, and we had formed a good personal relationship.

As back-up quarterback there, I would simulate an upcoming opponent's offense in practice so that Quinn's defense could prepare for a particular game day, and we grew close. I think he saw the hard work I put in for the squad as a whole and respected my efforts, while seeing up close that I was a good player.

When I walked into their practice facility, I was greeted by Dan like an old friend. It was great to see him and his smiling face, and I immediately could tell that he had brought so much of the Seahawks' energy with him. On the wall there was a big sign, a sign copied and posted all over the building. It read "BROTHERHOOD", and as I met the players and staff, it was clear that it was more than just a motto.

Dan himself pulled me to the side before the tryout and quietly told me that he was going to sign me, but it would be as a receiver, and he just needed me there that day to check and see if I was in good enough shape. I was, and I made the team, and it was so cool that he had so much faith in me from the start. Yes, I know I was signed at receiver, but that didn't matter. Not now, not with what my family was going through, with the grief we all shared for my grandmother and the fight we were all supporting my sister in.

My experiences in Chicago, being overwhelmed by emotion, how uncomfortable I had felt back in Tallahassee, it all made me just want to play and provide for my family, so being at receiver was fine with me. At that point, the regular season was coming to an end, and the team was playing well, with great players such as Matty Ryan at quarterback and Julio Jones at wide receiver. So, I knew I wouldn't get my feet on the field right away, but I loved being in Atlanta.

It was perfect. It was the closest I'd ever been to home with a team, which meant I was on the same time zone as my family and therefore in constant touch. Of course, not all our conversations were easy. My dad, a fierce competitor himself, knew firsthand how determined I had always been to play at quarterback.

This was a man who would get mad while playing catch with me because, as a kid, I would always overthrow a ball to him, forcing him to walk and pick it up, or I would throw it over a wall and lose it altogether, just to show him what a strong arm I had. Now, I was telling him that I was happy to play elsewhere, with a peace in my voice that he was mistaking for me giving up.

That wasn't the case at all, but when I phoned home, there was often the same talk. "Are you sure? Have you talked to the coach? Come on, son, you have the ability to play there." It got to the point where I had to set my dad straight. I was fine with not playing at quarterback in Atlanta, and frankly, it wasn't helping to listen to his disappointment because that was not my reality.

Instead, I was going to work happy, giving it my all every day, knowing that it would not be enough to get me on the team immediately, but still putting in the hard yards. They had even moved me to running back, which put me further down the totem pole because I had to learn to block the big guys and all that comes with that.

I was in the discussion, though, being thought about among a great set of players by a very good set of coaches, many of whom have gone on to become head coaches in their own right. It was a great place to be, made even better by the fact I had recently seen and felt what it was like to not be in it at all.

I didn't ever think that it was now or never at the Falcons, but I knew the clock was ticking, especially when one of the coaches alluded to my age – while not saying it directly, he implied that I was getting old. Twenty-six and time was passing me by, and I needed to take the game more seriously. That's what he said. It kind of upset me, especially considering the work I was putting in.

It didn't grate me for long, though. My time in the game had humbled me. The glory of the NFL is great – it's what makes it a global phenomenon. When it comes to putting on a show, nothing is quite like it, and even today, as I watch every week, I continue to love that aspect of the game. However, back then, in Atlanta, it dawned on me that there was so much more within it.

I look at the top athletes of my time across all sports, men like LeBron James, who continues to show an incredible thirst for glory. Every season, every week, every day in practice, people like LeBron, and so many more who haven't achieved his level of fame, come to work with a desire to succeed. That's something the fans don't see: the drive to go again, even when, like LeBron, you have achieved so much. The outside voices will find the nerve to knock someone like him if, say, he doesn't win a championship one year, but they only underline how little they know about pro sports.

Showing up and working hard to achieve things with teammates, wanting to be the best, accepting both success and defeats and going again – I never fell out of love with the game, and I learned to love the process. Practice was my playground. I loved going into work, figuring things out, and the peace I found at this time in my life brings me as much joy and pride as the Super Bowl ring that I own. I was working hard, I was getting paid a decent check, and that was helping with my sister's far more important experience with cancer.

Don't be mistaken, though. I was not some buddy-buddy new teammate coming onto the team, into the practice squad, simply to help the regular players get ready for game day. I was there to work, to be better than whoever was in my way, and I was there to take care of business in practice. My aim was to make the active roster, so in practice I was playing like I would in a game. I wasn't doing much smiling there. There was no laughing. I needed to find out the quickest way to earn respect, and that was to play like an aggressive dog.

My bark was there from the start. I was blocking hard, I was making hits with the intention of burying people in the ground. And I expected the same back because I wanted to show I could handle it. This was a great group, they lived by their "BROTHERHOOD" motto, but I was not there to make friends. As I saw it, if I was making friends, I was getting one step closer to a job at Walmart, and that was not happening.

Did I rustle some feathers? Yes, I did, and I was glad about it. Some of the coaches thought I was playing too strong, hitting their star players with too much determination. "BJ, you're going in too hard," they'd say. "Ease up, BJ." It was just like elementary school again when my teachers told my parents, "He plays too hard." My dad didn't listen to them then, and I certainly wasn't going to listen now.

Anyway, maybe it did those players some good to have me play so hard on them, because in the new year, they got through the playoffs and went to the Super Bowl. I was going back to Houston with them for a showdown, once again with the New England Patriots. This was my third experience of the game's finale, and the group could also draw on the knowledge I had gained.

Even in the playoffs, I was useful. There we faced the Seahawks, and Coach Quinn used me to help prepare the team, because he knew that I had an extensive knowledge of how their offense would play. They relied on those opinions, and in practice he would ask me to play and replicate my old teammate Russell Wilson.

That made me laugh to myself. I am a competitor, and that means I will never simply stand down and say that someone is better than me. Michael Jordan, he is the greatest basketball player, arguably the greatest athlete, of all time, but come the day that he plays against me, he is going to have to prove it. I will give him flowers when they're due, but if Michael is facing me on the court, he needs to bring it and show me up right then and there.

So, when I was asked to be Russell, the player I was backup to for so long, I found that hard. We did have many similar attributes, but I was signed to the Hawks as BJ Daniels, so I just wanted to be me. Whoever I was, it worked – the Seahawks were beaten, and those practices helped get the Falcons all the way.

Beating the Seahawks, going back to Houston, taking on the Patriots who had rejected me, it felt like the universe was constantly putting me back in the faces of those who had doubted me. It had happened to me ever since middle school, and with the belief I have in God, I took great strength in Him. The Bible tells us to be faithful and stay faithful, and if you believe, God will turn things around for you and make your enemies your footstool.

I took a lot from those words, and always tried to stay faithful to what I was doing. I stayed the course, and because of the fact that I kept working and treating people right, those opportunities would arise. Look, a lot was thrown at me – injuries, lots of obstacles put in my way – but through faith in God and myself, I was able to be elevated and experience these great moments. The tables will turn. Maybe not as quickly as you want them to, but with work and faith in yourself, they do, and when they do, it is thrilling.

I wanted to cuss people out, get mad, all the things natural to human beings. Throughout my athletic career, that seemed the natural thing to do, but by being calm, waiting, at school, college and in the pros, that elevation came, and it always felt better than any confrontation could.

Back in Houston, for the Super Bowl, I was very much involved, helping the running backs, going out prior to the game and throwing around with them. I very much enjoyed the occasion. My family had managed to come out, and as the game started, it seemed that our team would prevail. The Falcons took a massive 21–3 lead into the locker-room, but nothing in this game is ever certain.

To watch the team lose, 34–28, from that position was tough. People wonder how, and firstly you have to say that the Patriots and Tom Brady were magnificent, but I did see some complacency creep in at halftime. The team, while not immature, did not, in my opinion, handle the occasion with maturity. The job was not finished at halftime, and while Lady Gaga played the halftime show, in our locker room, there was not enough aggression.

When the Seahawks came in at halftime during the 2014 Super Bowl, 22–0 up, the mentality was, "Let's beat these guys to a pulp." The ambition was to not let them score at all. With the Falcons, I witnessed happiness. Don't get me wrong, it's good to be happy, but there was a comfort that I think weakened the team.

THE STRUGGLE TO SURVIVE

It wasn't all about halftime; some of the tactics in the second half didn't work for the team. They probably could have run the ball more, and in time, as the tide changed, all the momentum went to the Patriots. It was like witnessing a slow death. To watch Brady chip away, little by little, to see it close up, you realize that that's how greatness is achieved. A five-yard pass here, a ten-yard pass there. They all turned the game his team's way and proved that greatness is not always about the showy Hail Mary, but a gradual pursuit that gets a team to where they need to be.

The game was lost, and I tried to use my experience of two Super Bowls – and the experience of both victory and defeat on the biggest stage – to help console my teammates. I watched them try to wrestle with momentum and shift it back their way, but sometimes the flow is just too strong. Leaving Texas, I thought about the year I'd had.

I thought about the hotel rooms, the tryouts, the rejections, the opportunities, the cuts, the grief for my grandmother, and the determination that my sister was now showing. It was all in my mind. Football is one thing, and momentum on the field of play sometimes simply can't be stopped, but as we traveled back to Atlanta, I felt a pride in myself and in my family, and I knew that we were starting to turn the tide.

11

A DREAM REALIZED

THIS IS NOT THE END

17

A DREAM REALIZED

THIS IS NOT THE END

I am walking along a highway in Atlanta, wearing a pair of shorts and a T-shirt. I've been walking for a while now. Thoughts are running through my mind, thoughts about life. Real life. I wonder if anyone has seen me. Here I am, making my way along a highway in another city that I hardly know, and tears are streaming down my face. I wonder what this has all been for. Everything I have been through, the journey I have been on, the places I have wanted to get to, and now I am traveling by foot to places I don't want to be. The cars roll by. If anyone looks closely, they will have seen a guy who once was on their city's football team, a guy who has won the Super Bowl, a guy who was recently with them at theirs, but a guy who now, covered in sweat and tears, is walking their streets, uncertain of where they might lead him...

***

On that night in Houston, from the sidelines as I watched Tom Brady's New England Patriots cement their comeback and take the Super Bowl from my team, the Falcons, I saw firsthand how powerful momentum can be. With Brady calling the shots, the Patriots not only grabbed it, but they ran with it until it was wrapped around our necks, suffocating the team until there was no fight left.

Momentum. It's a game's most valuable asset. If a team gets control of it, it can be almost impossible to grab back. The same can be said for careers. As I stood there and watched both the celebrations of the winners and the devastation among my teammates, I thought about both sides of that coin. Throughout my career, I had witnessed both glory and defeat, but at that moment, while I still hoped to have a future with the Falcons, it crossed my mind that maybe I, or my career, had also lost the momentum. Was it impossible to grab back? I was about to find out.

I had actually enjoyed the experience in Houston. Not the final score, of course – that hurts to this day – but I was so young when the Seahawks won the Super Bowl in 2014, so I rode the wave of glory without fully appreciating any of it. This time felt different. I could stand back and take it in. In New York, I was looking to my left, looking to my right, and saying to myself, "Wow, this is so cool."

In Houston, there was perspective. I appreciated myself, was proud of how far I'd come. I remember reflecting on the fact that, in the almost four years I'd been in the NFL, I was part of three of the most memorable Super Bowls of the decade, if not the 21st century. That night, there were no clubs or late-night drinks, just some food at the hotel with my family, enjoying their company. The younger guys might have gone out – I would have if I was their age – but to be with my loved ones (including Laurel, whose cancer treatment was underway) was all I wanted.

The following season at Atlanta promised to be an interesting one for me. Although I had been practicing with the team as a wide receiver, Coach Quinn let me know that he wanted to switch me to running back. As I said before, I felt a newfound willingness to play wherever they put me, so I spent the offseason and summer preparing myself and turning into what I needed to be.

That meant getting into the gym, hitting the weight room harder than ever before, changing my diet, changing my body. Every meal was like a training session. I would sit down, and I'd be thinking about how much protein I was getting. I was training six days a week, and I went from 212lbs to 230lbs in just a few months.

It was necessary. I had gone from throwing the football, to catching and running with it, to now running and blocking for my quarterback and taking regular hits. My body had to be ready, and so did my mind. But, as it turned out, I had been too focused on the former, and with all the work I did to bulk up and improve my upper body strength, I had ignored my core. It was a mistake I would come to regret.

During training camp that summer, I suffered what is called a sports hernia, a gradual tear of the lower abdomen. It wasn't one incident that caused it; it was damaged over time, thanks to that weakened core that was supposed to hold everything together while I pushed myself to the limit. It was taking me longer to reach maximum speeds, there was no explosion in my running, and then, in time, I could not run at all. I could not engage my core or push away. There was no denying it – not only was I going to have to sit out at training camp, but I was going to have to go away and get surgery.

The Falcons released me, and my thoughts turned to the younger and fitter guys they would bring in to replace me. I understood that they had to cut me and replace me with a fitter guy, but as the general manager told me, once I got myself healthy, they would put me back on the squad. I went away determined to make that moment come around as quickly as possible.

Going away meant a trip to Philadelphia to see Dr. William Myers, a specialist in sports hernias and a doctor visited regularly by NFL and NBA players. The operation, paid for by the NFL, was a success, but I had to stay there, alone in a hotel, keeping my body elevated, and doing very little walking or moving.

So, as always, I found myself in another hotel room. As I ordered room service and watched the movies on TV, I wondered how many of these rooms I'd been in, and how many more I'd see as an NFL player. My body had just been opened up and stitched back together. I would soon be asking it to go again, to get back to battle. Was that asking too much of myself physically? And what about mentally?

My body responded well, healing nicely, and in months I was healthy, back in Atlanta – I had stayed there with my girlfriend – just waiting on the call to come back to the Falcons. The phone call never came. I had stayed in the city, watched every game from home, supported the team, feeling their pain as they lost in the playoffs, and with each game that passed by, it was becoming clearer and clearer that, despite their promise to bring me back once I was healed from the injury, my time with them was over. There would be no second chance.

So, there we were: my girlfriend and I, in Atlanta, me with decisions to make, her with a job and wondering what those decisions might be. What was clear to me, there and then, with that phone staying silent, was that I needed to get a job. So, I started a job hunt, and soon enough, I got an interview at a marketing firm.

It turned out to be a strange but important day. On the morning of the interview, I decided to walk to the office. It was pretty far away, and I had a car, gas, and money for more gas, but I just had this urge to test myself. I wanted to see if I could push myself in the ways that I had with football, so I packed my suit in a backpack, put on some shorts and sneakers, and headed out.

I wanted to test that injury, test my mind, so I walked along sidewalks, through industrial and construction sites, and even a small forest until I finally arrived. I went into the bathroom, freshened up, put on my suit, fixed my hair, and headed up before being told to sit and wait with another 15 people until my name was called.

When it was, I headed into the interview room, introduced myself, and began to answer their questions while telling my story. The guy interviewing me, his jaw hit the floor. I told him

I used to play for the Falcons, I was on their Super Bowl team. He couldn't believe it. He started to ask me questions about the NFL, about Marshawn Lynch and Odell Beckham. Then, he brought in his boss, who was equally as stoked by me and my recent past, and there and then they offered me the job. Could I start on Monday?

They took me around the office, introducing me to coworkers as BJ, a former Falcon, and when I left, I walked through the waiting room and could hardly look at the seven or so people waiting their interviews, knowing that, without answering many questions, I had the job that they were there for.

I went back to the bathroom, packed up my suit, put on my shorts and sneakers, and started my walk home. That's when I started to lose it. Overcome with emotion as I walked along the roads and highways, a mixture of sadness at what wasn't happening in my football career, and anger at how easy getting that job was. I thought about that joke in NFL locker rooms about doing what you're told or you'll end up working at Walmart, and all the things we had always been told to do. Change your position, change your body, change your diet, be this, be that – all these things started to rage through my mind.

I had walked to an interview, gotten the job, and I was walking home, things that people do every day, but as I continued to cry for all the rage I felt for the NFL, I was mourning the loss of it in my life. I wondered if people saw me as they drove past. Maybe I was anonymous enough in the city, but if they had, would this former athlete now crying on the sidewalk become the next social media meme?

A DREAM REALIZED

After a while, I called my girlfriend, who came and picked me up, and as we drove back to my apartment, she couldn't understand why I had walked or why I was so upset. We argued, and she dropped me home and drove away. She was tired of football being on my mind. She hoped that it was now in my past, and that it could finally just be me and her. I couldn't think like that.

Football was not in my life, but that wasn't by choice. I was still firmly clinging to the game, but I was being forced to move on with my life, and that is hard to take. I would do it, of course I would – I had just gotten a job with minimal effort – but my feelings of wanting to be playing somewhere wouldn't just disappear overnight.

As she drove away, I knew that I was done with Atlanta. I wouldn't be showing up to that job. On Monday, they called me, but I just ignored it. They emailed me, and I never replied. I completely blew it off. They must have wondered what happened to me, and if they are reading this, I apologize, but the job just wasn't for me. I was going home.

***

Back in Florida, while considering my next move, I wasn't going to simply forget the game. Opportunities were out there – they were, in some cases, obscure and even a bit demeaning, but they were to be seen as springboards back to where I wanted to be. With that in mind, I headed to the beautiful town of Vero Beach, Florida, where a competition program named *Your Call Football* gave me the chance to play, and hopefully get noticed.

Your Call Football was a strange phenomenon. We would play games, televised games, and the audience would, like in live betting, vote for the next play. The coach on the side would get the voting numbers and pass on the information to me at quarterback, and the audience's chosen play would be our next move.

I have to say, there were times I didn't agree with their calls, so, let's put it this way, I improvised. That would get me in trouble with the higher-ups who didn't like my free thinking. The whole set-up was kind of funny to me, but at the end of the day, I was in uniform, and I was throwing a football, both at games and in the training camp that went with it.

It wasn't long before I got a call from Canada. The Canadian Football League (CFL) is an interesting league, and one that I saw very much as the springboard back to the NFL that I was looking for. The Saskatchewan Roughriders, based in the city of Regina, were one of the strongest teams, and when they asked me to try out, I was not going to say no to the opportunity. For the first time in my life, I was leaving the country to play football.

Leaving the country meant leaving my family behind, and it also meant leaving my relationship behind. I didn't see it like that, of course – I saw it as a necessary move to get back into the league. But being with someone when you're an athlete means you have to ask a lot of them – it is far from a normal way of life. I was a football player, and I wasn't done yet. This time, though, the move was too much. We broke up, and I headed over the border alone.

And, as you probably guessed by now, my move to Canada was not easy. First of all, things were a little bit different up there. The field would be up to seven yards wider, and the end zone was ten yards bigger there. Plus, the teams play 12 vs. 12. It makes sense if you consider that the field is bigger: the extra man somewhat negates the extra space. I also found that, in the CFL, skill levels were far lower than in the NFL, but I was not looking down on any of it. I knew I'd have to fight to make the team.

Interestingly, CFL rules state that a team can only have a certain number of Americans on their roster, so with several Americans trying to make the season's squad, I might have been better than, say, 60 percent of the Canadians, but it was the Americans who were competing for the spots.

I was there to try out as a quarterback, and I was told back in Florida that the opportunity was for me to compete to be the starter. Once again, that was false information, but I was used to proving myself, and even in another country, I just put my head down and got to work.

The thing was, the team already had a starting quarterback, a Canadian, and *he* was competing for the spot with a backup guy, a Canadian Super Bowl winner. When the Roughriders signed the latter quarterback, they gave him a contract that made him the highest-paid player in the entire league. So, I was coming in as backup to both of those guys. As I said, it would not be easy.

But, grateful to be there, I got to work, going hard in practice, learning the playbook, throwing really well and getting along with the guys in the locker room. I liked it because most of the players up there had a story. The American guys were mostly like me: either looking for a way back into the NFL, or just desperate to play. Often, it was a little bit of both.

They were interested in my story too, the Super Bowl win, of course, and I enjoyed both their company and the competitiveness of practices there. I had always loved the fire that burns when there is something to prove, and this was a field full of guys with the same motive. I was playing great, even though I was unhappy with the line of highly paid players who had been put in front of me without my prior knowledge, but I put that disappointment into practicing hard and hoping to get my chance to prove what I could do.

When the preseason came around, I was only getting what is known as "garbage time" on the field, playing right at the end of the games. In the second game, I got to call only eight plays. The last of them, I made my pass, but the receiver ran right, when I thought he was running left. The pass was intercepted, they took me out of the game, and right there and then, I knew they were done with me. I was right.

I only made 8 plays out of the 78, but with that one interception, in came the judgment. It didn't strike me as athletically correct. One strike and you were out? Was that how it worked? The best players, the Bradys and the Mannings, they were allowed to make mistakes, I got that, but it didn't seem that the rest of us got the same grace.

Sports should be about examining how competitors react to mistakes. For example, boxing is a test of how hard a fighter can get hit and still persevere. In basketball, if a player misses a lay-up, they don't get benched immediately – they get the chance to shoot the ball again on the next play.

A DREAM REALIZED

For me, and guys like me trying to prove themselves, such luxuries did not apply. Life might be about second chances, but football wasn't, unless you were already right at the top. If you're thinking, *That doesn't sound fair*, you're damn right it wasn't. I had thrown one pass, a bad one, even if the receiver had made the wrong run. That was all on me, and that was that.

So, I was going back to Tallahassee, and I hadn't made it into the CFL. If it had been hard to come home having been cut from the NFL, this took me to an even darker place. No job, back at my parents' place in my old bedroom, deemed not good enough for the Canadian league. My ego and my dreams were both broken. As I said, I never once looked down at the CFL, but being told "no, thanks" by a team up there was always going to hurt.

Back in my hometown, my mind drifting, my ego battling against what was happening to me, I couldn't help but think that I had played in football's top league, was with the country's top teams, but in my keenness to keep playing the game, I had traveled down into the valley, and even down there, they didn't appreciate me.

It felt like my options were running out, and as I made my way around the city in which I grew up, the feelings I had as a kid, of wanting to be different, to see the world, they would not go away. But I wondered how I would be able to do that now – I had always thought that I would see and do the things I wanted through football.

I wanted to fly on planes, I wanted to see different cities, meet new people, and it was through the game that those dreams had been at least partially realized. Now, with so many doors being closed, I felt like I was destined, like so many of my high school peers, to stay, live and die in my hometown. Again, to be clear, I am not mocking that, it's just that I always wanted more. Football might have been in my future anymore, but I still wanted to achieve so much.

When I was young, one of the chores I disliked most was helping my mom in the backyard. She loves to grow things, and she would have me help out. Mom had grown up in a rural setting, and she loves nature.

I was the opposite: I craved concrete, high buildings, the big city – life outside of the backyard. Now, only in my late 20s, the idea that it was time to put my gardening gloves back on and resume a quiet life was not sitting right with me. There was still a lot for me to do, I knew that much. In the short term, though, I needed a job, and as luck would have it, someone very close to me was hiring.

At that time, my dad had been coaching the girls' basketball teams at Leon High School for 16 years. As it turned out, he could do with an assistant, and because of my knowledge of elite sports and training methods, he made me strength-and-conditioning coach. Talk about a humbling experience. Even with all the things that had happened after Atlanta – the end of my relationship, seemingly the end of my football career – it was hard to believe that I was living at home and working under my dad, coaching teenage girls' basketball.

But as it turned out, I absolutely loved the job. Having spent weeks and months since leaving the Falcons chasing

A DREAM REALIZED

a football dream, I found myself coming to work with a new gusto. It was so fulfilling, far more than I expected. To be able to pass on knowledge, to be able to have these young people listen and take in what I had learned, that was special. I was their motivator, and I was able to push them beyond their limits.

Young people can be like a blank canvas. They don't know just how much they can achieve, they don't know what they can and can't do, so, with the right guidance and backing, so much can be done. Basketball is far more physical than some people think, and because of my time as football player, I could teach them about the conditioning that would help them run and jump while absorbing contact. I did that, and they listened, and then they succeeded. I loved it.

If anything, the biggest obstacle I faced in the job came in the shape of my boss. It was great working closely with my dad, but it must have been strange for him, having done his job alone for so long, and then to have me, his son, suddenly bringing all these new ideas to the students. My dad and I, we have similar personalities. We're both Scorpios (if you are into that), and we're both competitors. So, my strong will to see these girls push themselves further than they had before, well, that might have taken some getting used to.

He was thinking of their best interests, not wanting to push them so hard that they failed, not wanting to ask too much. We never fought about it, of course, but we did have some intense conversations about what was actually best for them. In the end, he did appreciate how much I was learning and the knowledge I brought. I guess there were times when his son was educating him a little bit – and that would probably be hard for any father to take.

Teaching and coaching seemed to come naturally to me. All the things I had looked for in my own teachers, those fantastic ones that not only teach but truly invest in their students – well, I was aspiring to be just like them. By the second year at Leon, I was assisting with the girls' basketball team *and* the boys' football team.

It was strange because when I was at Lincoln, Leon were our biggest rivals. We hated each other. Those games meant so much, and I have to say, when I was playing, Lincoln would always win. I think there was a 27-game winning streak, and I relished the ones I was involved in. Yes, I used to beat that team every year, but now I was at Leon, trying to help the team turn the tables.

Although I had somewhat butted heads with my dad, the differences in opinion were a little bit more intense with the football head coach. I think I threatened him because I could really use my football knowledge and hands-on experience to teach the kids about the game. I knew how they could learn the playbook, lift weights, improve their footwork and perform intricate maneuvers, like the three-step drop. It was clear though that the coach didn't want any of that. He was after an assistant who would do only what the job title said: assist. That meant following his lead.

I certainly wasn't there to upset anyone. The community knew me, as did the kids, and I understood that might get in his way. Instead, I figured out a way to serve the players in some other capacity, and that meant being the guy they could lean on. I was there for them, an ear to hear their problems at school or at home. If they came off the field mad or upset, I was there to listen, talk and offer encouragement.

I learned not to focus on the intricacies of the game I loved, but on the kids themselves. It was hard, but I began to love it. By humbling myself, I realized that the feelings I had felt since my grandmother and sister's illnesses, those feelings of wanting to take all I had experienced in the game of football and use it to help others, that could become something very real.

Having said all that, there was still the pull of football, and I couldn't resist when football and a chance to play it at a good level came along. This time it was a team in Salt Lake City, the Stallions, playing in the Alliance of American Football League. I was instantly interested.

The AAF was played in the spring, so having finished the high school season with Leon, and having been drafted by the Stallions, I was off to Utah. The head coach there was a guy named Dennis Erickson, a brilliant man, a college football Hall of Famer who worked with the Miami Hurricanes and had won national championships. Both Florida men, we hit it off. Meanwhile, there was another familiar face on the team, but this one was going to cause me problems.

The same guy who had been brought in by the New York Giants when I was there, the guy they cut me for, before letting him go and asking me back, well, he was with the Stallions too. We were both picked, but he had been picked first, so I was going to have to oust him once again if I wanted to start.

That didn't bother me. I had stayed in good shape, my coaching had kept my arm strong, and I already knew that my knowledge was superior to his. If everything went well, I would make the team ahead of him. But, as this story has taught us, everything rarely goes to plan.

I was driven by my desire to play. I liked the league's structure, the pay was decent, the games were televised, it offered great exposure, and the people in it seemed sincere and shared my passion. All my focus was on one thing: becoming the Stallions' starting quarterback. In the preseason, I made a pass in the second game, got tackled, and as I put my left arm out to break my fall, something snapped. *Pop.* I knew it was fairly bad, but it being my left arm, I played on, taking the snap with one hand, and then, two plays later, calling a shotgun and throwing a touchdown pass.

I then left the field so they could look at the other guys, and when the medical team examined me, it turned out that I had torn my bicep away from the elbow tendon. Without help, I wouldn't play anytime soon. I was so desperate to be out there that I began to contemplate any option – even illegal ones.

I inquired about steroids. That's how much I wanted it. What was the quickest way of getting me back out there? The quickest, not the safest, and even with the threat of long-term damage to my body and the peril of possible drug testing, I seriously considered injections. Why not? I had already done everything that was asked of me. I put in the hard work. I studied to get grades good enough

A DREAM REALIZED

to get me into college because that's what I was told to do. I listened to everything, followed along, all for my dream, and now this. Why shouldn't I do all I could, by any means necessary?

In the end, I couldn't bring myself to damage myself and my reputation in that way. Instead, I had another surgery, opened my body once again in the name of my dream. But there was something different this time – because Coach Erickson believed in me as a player and a person, instead of cutting me or sending me home with false promises that I'd be back on the roster, he actually kept me around.

To other coaches, I might have been damaged goods, unable to contribute, easily offloaded and replaced by someone young and strong, but not to Coach Erickson. For the first time in my career, here was someone who saw beyond my injury and felt that even if I was unfit to play, my knowledge and ability as a veteran and leader could help his team. He was a coach who believed in me. That was special. I couldn't wait to get healthy again and repay him. However, in April 2019, the league ceased operating for financial reasons, so I never got the chance. Instead, I was once again making the journey back to my hometown.

Work-wise, there was another football season to coach at Leon, but then my phone rang. This time it was *another* league, the XFL, a professional minor league. The team that wanted me was in, of all places, Seattle. As soon as I stepped off the plane, I felt a wave of love from the city that had already given me so much.

It was February 2020, and the Seattle Dragons needed a back-up quarterback to cover a guy named Brandon Silvers, who was their starter. There was no anger on my part, no disillusion in being asked to cover a first-string quarterback. This was an opportunity, a chance to do what I loved. I respected that chance more than ever, and as a 30-year-old man among mostly younger guys, some just out of college, some away from home for the very first time, I was more than happy to be a support system, if they wanted one.

One thing I did was start a prayer and study group. It was a space for the guys to come and discuss anything that was on their minds, whether it had to do with football or not. We talked about financial literacy, we talked about how to treat people, we talked about standing up for what you believed in and for yourself, and about how, sometimes, the coach really doesn't know best. They were great sessions, ones that I hope helped some of my teammates. I know they helped me.

During the second-to-last game of the season, against the St. Louis Battlehawks, our starting quarterback wasn't playing very well, so they took him out and sent me in. Just like that, I was a ball of energy. It was like I was back in high school, taking the field in front of college scouts, as if the rest of my career depended on it. I played well and was interviewed afterward on TV. I simply said that I was grateful to be given the opportunity to be there, and that was the truth.

After I played so well against St. Louis, the coach decided to put me in for the final game of the season against the Houston Roughnecks. I was starting. I was a starting

A DREAM REALIZED

quarterback, and when I threw the first touchdown of the game, an overwhelming sense of gratitude and satisfaction came over me. It was very similar to the touchdown I had scored with the Chicago Bears that had brought so much joy to my grandmother before she passed. This game meant very little in the grand scheme of sports, but to me, it meant so much. To be there, starting and throwing touchdowns, it brought such clarity to everything, making every struggle seem suddenly worth it.

Just weeks later, though, the world stopped. The Covid-19 pandemic took hold of the planet, and while no one knew how long that hold would last, sports, like everything else, were suspended. As we all know now, they would be shut down for a long, long time, and so that was that. My pro football career was over. I guess you could say it took a global pandemic to stop me.

The XFL. It doesn't sound like much, but to be in that moment, for that last game, everything that I ever wanted was realized. It was every aspiring young football player's dream of what it would be like to get into the NFL. I remember when I was sitting in my parents' bathroom and hanging up the phone after getting drafted by the 49ers. I thought I had made the dream come true. But the thing I know now is that the dream isn't getting to the NFL – it's *playing* in it.

I am going to die one day, and sometimes I reflect on that and think that I might have finished my career without ever starting at quarterback as a pro athlete. All that I went through, all that I saw, the surgeries I endured, the setbacks

I overcame, if I had never started as a pro, how could I have said it was worth it?

That's what the itch was. That's what made me travel the length of the country and beyond. All the Super Bowl rings in the world meant nothing next to that goal. I wanted to start, and then, for a team in Seattle, a city that meant so much to my story, it happened. And not only that, but I had excelled.

When people think of sports, their minds understandably turn to glory and trophies. Players at the start of their careers think of bowl games, the rings, the yards they will make or stop, and the Hall of Fame. I was the same, but then I realized something more was at stake: my dreams. And finally, they had come true. It was over now, but I could go home happy. I had peace.

12

MY FAITH

WHERE I FIND SUPPORT AND COMFORT

But by the grace of God, I am what I am, and his grace to me was not without effect. No, I worked harder than all of them — yet not I, but the grace of God that was with me.
Corinthians 15:10

When I was young — not even ten years old, I don't think — my dad took me to my baseball team's end-of-season summer barbeque. It was being held at our coach's house, and all the players and their parents were there. The kids were in full uniforms, there to enjoy a summer afternoon, be proud of ourselves and our team, and enjoy the many hot dogs coming off the grill.

We all gathered outside by my coach's swimming pool, and everything seemed to be going great. I was very young, but I sensed that my dad, usually so accommodating and accepting of people, was not a big fan of this guy. There was always a silence when he was talked about, and my dad certainly wasn't ever making any kind of effort be around him or to get close to him.

I liked being on the team. I loved baseball in the summer, and as a kid, I just saw the coach as an adult, an authority figure, one that I had to respect. Even if his behavior around me was slightly strange.

I was the only Black kid on the team, a fact that never bothered me. I was just me. Because of sports, I mixed with all different people from a young age, so different skin colors didn't really mean anything to me. The coach, however, would make jokes, ones that I would pick up on now, but I didn't then. Plus, whenever he talked to me, he would turn his baseball cap backwards. I thought, probably naively, that he was just trying to relate to me. It was a strange dynamic, but at his house that day, all I cared about was playing with my friends and having more ketchup on my hotdogs.

But then it happened. As I was walking past the swimming pool, the coach walked toward me, picked me up – fully clothed with my shoes still on – and threw me in. I could not swim, and I don't know if he knew that or why he would do that to me, but without warning, I found myself sinking to the bottom of the pool, without any knowledge of how to get back to the surface.

Before I could truly panic, my dad was down there with me, his clothes on too, his cellphone ruined in his pocket, taking me in his arms and pulling me back up. We climbed out of the pool and started to ring out our clothes while the whole party stood there, staring at us.

I remember feeling ashamed, like I had caused a scene. All I wanted to do was get back to hanging out with my teammates. But my dad, quietly furious over what had just happened, had other ideas. I could see he was mad enough to try and lay his hands on this guy, so we left. Driving home, he tried to console me, telling me that some people are different, some people's cultures are different, but that this coach's behavior was not acceptable or normal in any way.

I was young. The idea that some people were different, that some people were not kind, and that some people would choose to do what that man had done to me, was new, and it generated new emotions in me.

Not long after that, I was sitting in our local Baptist church. I can't recall a time in my life when the church has not been part of my or my family's life. My dad is a deacon and was very much involved in the church. Every Sunday that I can remember from my childhood, we would be there. I would wear a suit, my dad would too, and my mom and my sisters would be in their best dresses. It was a constant, a place where our community came together.

So, as my age turned to double digits, and I started dealing with new emotions, like the ones I experienced after being thrown into the pool, I could always rely on my family, but I also always had my church. I spent all of my Sundays there.

At the end of the service, they always asked if anyone there would like to stand up and give their life to God. If anyone wanted to make a declaration to God. I'm not sure how it happened, but one Sunday, without feeling any pressure or being forced, I looked up to my dad and I said, "Dad, I want to do it. I want to give my life to God." My dad smiled, and said, "Go ahead." So, there I was, a ten-year-old boy walking up the aisle on my own, everyone looking at me. When I got to the preacher, he asked me if I believed,

I nodded, and he asked if I would like to be baptized. I nodded again. A couple of Sundays later, I was.

From that young age, I felt compelled to be part of something, to be part of the church. While those emotions I'd felt when my baseball coach threw me into the water were new and confusing, being baptized could not have felt clearer.

From that point on, I took lessons from church and have always tried to live my life by its teachings, but part of that is accepting people's flaws, maybe even that baseball coach's. Because of what I've learned at church, I try to not judge people, and instead accept people as they are. Yes, they might let me down eventually, but I must allow them into my community and offer them a chance. Love and trust: both go a long way.

When I was playing, I became close friends with very different kinds of people. Take Marshawn Lynch and Russell Wilson at the Seahawks. You could not find two more different guys, two individuals from totally different walks of life. I was and am close to both. I took them as they came, finding a way to be myself with both, treating them as the church taught me. Starting on an even playing field is the best way to begin.

Today, I talk to a lot of people. I may be giving talks to young adults, supporting a student one-on-one, or approaching a CEO in my job as a fundraiser at USF. These are people of all ages and from both sides of the tracks. I always try to relate to the person in front of me. I can go into an elementary school, a college or a Fortune 500 corporation's

MY FAITH

office, and find ways to communicate with my audience that will resonate with them.

When I was a quarterback, I had to be able to talk to each member of that team. He might have been a guy from rural Ohio, or he might have been from Compton, but all I knew was that he was with me, and we had to communicate together and work as one. Now, when I talk to these different people today, the same thing applies, and my ability to hopefully be able to do that, it all comes from my family, my church and my faith.

By having the values that my church and my faith have taught me, and taking them into the wider community and beyond, I have found it easier to truly get to know people. If someone comes to me at USF with a problem, I want them to feel comfortable because what they're doing is not easy. I'll thank for them for trusting me with their problem and I will look for a story from my life that's relatable, in order to show them that I have made many mistakes, problems are part of our lives, and everyone can make it through them.

I may be wearing a suit, be in an office, they may see memorabilia on the shelves from my football career, but I don't want them to think that I am some sort of all-conquering ex-athlete who has broken through life's brick walls without a scratch. That is far from who I am, and in time, they get to understand me, and that my story is all about imperfection. And that's more than okay.

To judge someone is to not understand someone. "He that is without sin among you, let him cast the first stone" is how Jesus put it, and in my working life and in that capacity trying to help young people and students, I try to remember that, and everything else the Bible teaches me. I never force my religion on anyone – I wouldn't do that. Instead, I carry it with me through my life and use it to guide me through situations and relationships.

I guess it has always been there. During my teenage years, with all those hormones raging and thought processes rebelling, my faith got a bit, let's say, blurred. I think that's normal, but then when I most needed it, I found it through the blur, and it became my strength once again.

Take my senior year of high school, when I wasn't getting any interest from schools, and there were no offers of full scholarships. My life seemed quite traumatic and dark, and I felt like I was losing my path. But my family and my faith were there for me. My dad asked me to write a list of all my goals, all the things that I wanted to accomplish. I did exactly that, and the truth is I did not accomplish a single one of them.

I wanted to be the best quarterback in the state. I wasn't. I was the second best. I wanted to win the State Championship. We didn't. But, by writing them down, and therefore believing that they might come true, things began to change, and with an attitude given strength by my belief in myself and my goals, schools began to turn their eyes on me. The great Nick Saban at Alabama, Michigan, Memphis – big schools, big names, who wanted to talk.

I, of course, went with USF. That's because of loyalty, something else I learned from church, and as South Florida had been the first to make me an offer, they were my first

MY FAITH

choice. With Jim Leavitt showing his own Christian values when he spoke and offering so much love at Keeley Dorsey's funeral, I instantly knew this was a university and a man I could play for. My faith would not have had it any other way.

During my career as an NFL player, and during those many months when I was chasing a place back in it, I am not sure how I could have coped without my faith. Sitting in those hotel rooms, waiting in those airport lounges, all by myself, my faith often gave me companionship. It still does. By leaning on it, those moments of potential loneliness are easily avoided.

Religion in sports is nothing new. You will see players making their way onto the field or onto the court, and they will pray to their god(s). I did, too. I would like to say that when I was young, I had wisdom, and when I prayed, I was asking for health, safety for me and those playing the game, for the strength to simply be my best. But really, I was praying to win. I think you'll find most players do the same.

As I say, most players are young, and with maturity, prayers and hopes mature, too. The things I ask for now have evolved. Winning, getting rich, glory – they have no place ahead of family, health, strength and protection, something I learned when my grandmother died and my sister Laurel got sick.

Living a life where you only want to win brings so much pressure and chaos with it. I've realized that my desire to find peace has simplified what I asked for in my prayers. I have also come to see that during my career, my belief in God was every bit as important to me and my performance as the weights I lifted and the practice I put in.

So, in my post-football life, the same things apply. I live my life and conduct myself at work with a belief and a faith that continues to grow and guide me. Recently, I have discussed with my dad the possibility of becoming more involved in the church. I have watched our preacher and felt an urge to do the same. I don't have the arrogance to think I could do it, but it feels like I should do it. We will have to see.

What I *can* say is, my story happened because of my faith. Belief creates opportunities, and I make the best of them with the strength that I take from God. I have not always succeeded, I have not always been the good man I should have been, but I did it all with faith, and with the grace of God that was with me.

13

LEAVE NO ONE BEHIND

FROM ATHLETIC DREAMS TO A LIFE PURPOSE

13

Having returned for a visit to Tallahassee, I went out one night with old friends from home. At that time, I was a Seattle Seahawks player. An NFL guy. So, I bought the drinks, told them some stories about who I was meeting, what my teammates were really like and what it felt like to have a Super Bowl ring. We hung out for hours, and at about two or three in the morning, we headed to a gas station to pick up something to eat.

Walking up to the station, there was a homeless man sitting in front of us, and as the others walked ahead, this guy's eyes locked with mine. Normally, in that split second, I would have thought that maybe the guy was going to ask for something, a bit of food from the store or a few dollars from my pocket. But this time, the thought was different. I immediately realized that we knew each other.

He was a guy I went to high school with, someone I had known well, a friend who I had played on the football team with and liked a lot. It had been several years since I had seen him, but I immediately recognized him and appreciated him. He had been my running back. He ran for me, he blocked for me, he laid his body on the line for the team, helping me to shine and be successful.

"Hey man," he said, clearly recognizing me too. "You're doing good. I've been following your career, BJ. You're doing real good." It was a humbling moment. And then I sensed embarrassment and shame from him. I didn't know his story, but standing there, all I felt was admiration, and then, for the first time, I felt bad for making it in football.

We stood, just for a couple of seconds, and then he walked away. I could have helped him, given him something, made his life a tiny bit easier, but he walked away. He didn't want anything from me. I never saw him again.

I stood there in silence. An hour or so before, I had been the life of the party, the hero who had returned to his hometown. But as my former high school teammate walked away into the darkness, I felt a change. I felt all those things that I was doing, all the athletic success that I was chasing, while it was so important to me, it was not and could not be everything.

I was just like that guy – I had been blessed with some talent – but I had made it through to the NFL. I realized then that my career couldn't define me, couldn't define who I was as a man. I was young, trying to make my way through life, but my life happened to involve athletic ambitions that others seemed to think put me on a pedestal. I was just like them, though: I experienced pain, I knew grief and disappointments, and I had to figure out ways to navigate this world and its darkest moments.

What I began to realize after that night was that I could share my experiences with people who might want to hear them, not for laughs or congratulations in some late-night bar, but to help them on their own journeys. After that, as my career moved forward and obstacles continued to change my path, that feeling grew and grew. I knew I would not have all the answers, I knew I was making mistakes as I went, but I also knew things were happening for a reason, and that, in time, I could somehow offer support.

***

In 2020, as the world tried to restart after pausing for Covid, my thoughts were very much on supporting myself. My football career was over – I had left the locker room as a player for the very last time – but I could still hear that NFL joke about working at Walmart in my head. This time, though, coming home no longer felt like a negative to me. The end of my football career happening along with the pandemic? It felt like something new had to begin, so home was probably the right place to be.

Because I had enjoyed my time coaching basketball and football at Leon so much, I knew that I wanted to get back on that path, and that perhaps it would eventually lead me back to the NFL. Coaching at the very top level was something I wanted back then, so I started to look for opportunities. One soon appeared, and it was on very familiar ground.

My two sisters, easily my two biggest fans, always championing and looking out for their big brother, let me know that they had seen a job posting from Lincoln High School, my old stomping grounds. They needed a new head coach for the football team. At first, we laughed about it, the idea of me going back there, the former quarterback, walking the halls, telling the kids what to do and how to act. However, with time, the more I discussed the possibility with family, there were fewer and fewer laughs. Soon, the idea didn't seem so crazy, so I applied, and I got an interview.

I went in unsure if I would get it. I had a decent resume, and I did well at Leon, but I had just turned 30, so I thought I was too inexperienced for the role of head coach. The school seemed to agree – they went with an older guy. I went in for three interviews, and felt I did well, but in the end, they went with a guy with more experience. They did say that they liked me, and although they chose to go in a different direction, they said that the other guy might want to hire me as an assistant.

That possibility interested me, but then I got another call from the high school, and it wasn't about the assistant job. It turned out that they'd had a change of heart. After comparing my interview with the other candidate's, they realized that they preferred more of my answers. So, they asked, would I consider accepting the head-coaching role? Normally, I probably would have asked why they didn't see me as the right man from the jump, but I was too excited for that conversation. This was a great opportunity, and I was going to take it and run with it. I was a head coach.

I was immediately thrown into the role, and I had so much to learn – quickly. I knew I could work with high schoolers, that was a given, and I knew I could reach them. It was the other stuff – dealing with their parents, the rosters, the budget, the equipment, the bus schedules – that's what took some getting used to. Once I did, though, we had a great football program.

The kids were good – Lincoln's players always had been. There were nationally ranked All-Americans on the roster. And now, they were being coached by an equally impressive staff. I had opened my contact book and very quickly brought in former NFL guys to work at the school, including first-round draft pick of the New York Jets, Calvin Pryor.

It was an incredible set-up, and results followed. Finding our feet, we lost a game, but then went on a winning streak (the season was shortened because of the pandemic) before we lost a game in the playoffs. In time, the entire community was talking about our program, and everyone wanted to come play at Lincoln.

It was a good time. Not only was the football program successful, but far more importantly, my sister Laurel was cancer-free just a year after her diagnosis. She was able to leave the hospital, ring that bell to tell the world that she had beaten the disease. For her, our family and everyone who loves her, the ringing of that bell was the most beautiful noise we'd ever heard. I am so proud of her. I am proud of both of my siblings.

Laurel also got her degree during Covid, which prevented her from having a huge ceremony, but we celebrated her, of course. I am constantly in awe of her and Eleana. The intensity and passion with which they selflessly serve their communities (Laurel as an elementary school teacher and Eleana as the director of player development and operations for the University of New Orleans women's basketball team) make them deserving of so much.

For me, after a season at Lincoln, I knew that the community I wanted to serve might be a little further away. My lifelong desire to go to other places kicked in, and when my alma mater, USF, asked for me to join their football team's coaching staff, it didn't take me long to pack my bags and move — for the second time in my life — from Tallahassee to Tampa.

I had gotten to know the head coach there, a guy named Jeff Scott. Being a high school coach, I had helped him with recruiting the kids at Lincoln. Now, I was one of his assistants, and coaching came naturally to me. The thought of going all the way to the NFL (again) seemed both possible and logical.

In time, though, such ambitions were checked. I loved working with the guys, but at this stage of my life, I felt that the sheer relentlessness of the job was too much. Football had been at the forefront of my mind since I was a kid, and the job, even at the college level, is an all-consuming, year-round commitment. And if the team's record slips, well, the *entire* coaching staff is out. I definitely gained, while doing that job, a newfound respect for all the guys I worked with.

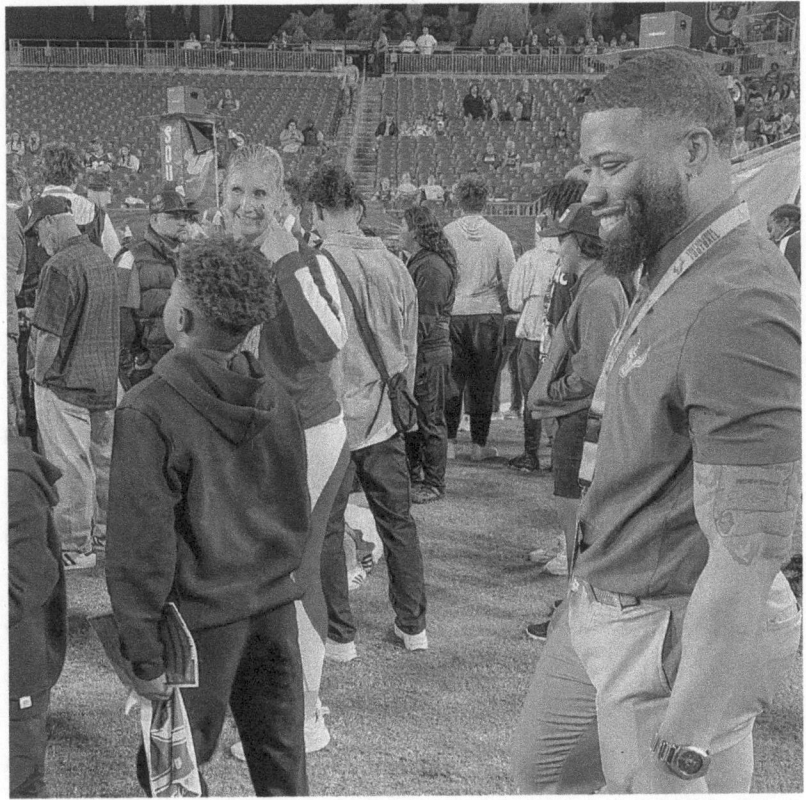

On the sidelines at USF

With that in mind, and with job security becoming something I wanted, I changed careers. In 2021 I made the move to USF's business wing, where I still work at the time of writing this book. I'm the Assistant Director of Donor, Community and Alumni Engagement in Development. I am also the head of the USF Athletics Alumni Association.

I may one day return to coaching, and I certainly will continue to work with the students and the football team, but for now I really enjoy my work, helping to build up the university and raising money for its athletic department. The job feels very natural to me. Maybe it's another success in my life that traces back to my younger days and that fire truck. If I want something enough, I'm going out hard to get it. When it comes to funds for these kids and their athletic ambitions, that fire truck *will* become a new skateboard.

Before I started the job, I had never asked anyone for money before, but when I approach large businesses and important people of commerce, I don't beg. What I want them to understand is that by donating money to university athletics, they are not giving money away – they are investing in people, young people who will serve the community in the future. I want these donors to see that they are getting something back for their money. They get to watch great sports, yes, but they also get to watch these young people grow. They have invested in them, and in time, they and the city of Tampa will reap the rewards.

I love my job, but that doesn't mean that I don't look out at the football field and miss it sometimes. Most ex-athletes will miss their former playground, and when I hear the laughter and camaraderie coming from the locker room, it takes me back to the time when my days were spent playing the game I love with my teammates, my brothers.

It's that feeling of missing football that makes me think I might return one day to coaching, but for now, I come into work, and those players know that my office door is always open, should they need to lean on me. They also know that I am in every day, working to better their student experience, and the experience of those who will attend USF in the future. In this role, I draw on so much from my time as a pro football player.

Take the way I dress at work. When I was a player, I would go into practice, and I would be dressed as if I was playing for a championship. Others might just put on the helmet, their pads, a pair of shorts, but not me. I was in full uniform. Tights, wristbands, matching gloves, all ready to go. I dressed for the job I wanted. So, at USF, you will find me, the only person in the department, wearing a suit – every day, tie on, the works. I look like I am the president of the university. Just like the football uniform, the suit is my armor now, and it tells others – and reminds me – that I've come to do my job.

When I go out to meet the CEO of a large company, or any other potential donors, that is like game day for me. I head to those meetings with all the drive I felt when I played football. And as I did during those times, I feel I have something to prove. I walk in knowing that I have to convince people. If they are going to give the university money, I, the face of that institution, have to assure them that they are making the right decision. It's nothing new. I have been trying to prove myself all my life. Now, with a university and people's futures at stake, it just means that much more.

***

I have felt for a long time that I can make a difference. Not only to the university's bank balance, but also to the people who study there, and anyone else trying to make their way in life. Mental health has long been a fascination of mine. Even as a young man, I wondered about my own feelings. When things got tough, I sensed that change, but I never knew how to put it into words.

Even growing up in the 1990s and into the 21st century, men of all ages didn't talk about feelings. Be tough. Get over it. Move on. In football it was all about taking the hits, getting up and going again. But my time in the game showed me that it is only through communication and teamwork that a person can truly make up the yards. That cannot be done alone.

There is a quote from a football legend that, for too long, I did not appreciate. Tony Dungy, a Hall of Fame coach, the first African American to lead a team to Super Bowl glory, once said, "Don't worry about your platform; focus on your impact."

For so long, I was consumed with where I was: the NFL. The platform in which I lived and played was everything. I loved the elevation it gave me, the fame, the glory, so much so that I forgot what I could do while up on that pedestal. Soon, when it was all over, I no longer had the NFL as my platform, but with Dungy's words in my heart, it no longer bothered me. I knew that I could still have an impact – and I found a way to do it.

It was when I became Lincoln High School's head coach that I first put Dungy's words into action. It was a Friday night that had turned into Saturday morning, and I was in the school's basement. It was cold and dark, and apart from the roaches, I was alone. I couldn't have been further away from the NFL than I was at that moment, but I didn't care about that. I had a job to do.

The team had played a game, and as coach, I made sure everyone had gotten home, and then, it was down to the basement to make sure the uniforms, both jerseys and pants, were washed and dried, ready to go again. They were sweaty, they did not smell good, and the job of cleaning them was on me. Who else was I going to ask?

Those nights down there, leaving in the early hours of the morning, not only did I garner a lot of satisfaction, but I knew that by silently doing my job, I was having an impact on those kids' lives, and that can mean so much more than a Super Bowl ring. My time as Lincoln's head coach happened years after I ran into my old running back at the gas station, a guy whose life clearly hadn't been easy, a guy who once wore the same football uniform as me. But even in the darkness of that basement, I realized that there was an impact that could be made. Help was out there. I realized that there was always hope and light.

Because of that realization, I have been able to meet so many people and work with new organizations, such as Shawmind, a mental health charity in the United Kingdom. Run by a friend, Adam Shaw, the charity pledges itself to young people everywhere, and our shared motto, "Leave No One Behind," resonates with and inspires me every day.

I work closely with the USF football team. I understand the guys' troubles, but that hope and that light extends to everyone. I have always lived my life with what I see as a healthy disrespect for authority. You may have noticed it within these pages. I think that people should be taken at face value, and whether they are the university's janitor or its president, they are the same, with their own problems, both sometimes in need of help, and both equally deserving of that help.

By working with Shawmind, a charity an ocean away, I know how far that help can stretch, so why not think these big thoughts like, *I want to help the world*? I've seen firsthand how far people can reach, people who look like me. When the Seahawks won the Super Bowl, the team and the staff were invited to the White House. As I kid, I never even thought I'd visit the nation's capital, let alone meet the President of the United States. It was a surreal day.

The team presented President Barack Obama with a jersey, and regardless of politics, for me to meet someone in the highest office in the country who looked like me, who might share some of my story, that was incredible.

We all got to greet him, and when we shook hands, I put my left arm on his shoulder. The Secret Service was all around us, so I could have gotten tasered, but then he reciprocated. Almost in an embrace, I said, "Man, it's a pleasure to meet you… like, seriously." Simple words, but then he looked back into my eyes. "I really appreciate that," he said. "Thank you."

Hardly a life-changing conversation to anyone listening, but for me, to witness close up how humble even the most powerful man on the planet could be, it underlined that it is the humanity that we share, not the positions that people hold, that is most important.

Today, my parents have the photo of that moment with me and the president up on a wall in their home. It is a snapshot from a life that would not have happened without their love, guidance and support. Everything that I achieved in sports is because of them being there, taking me to each practice and game. Because of their words of wisdom, I kept moving forward, even when it didn't seem possible. But now, it is because of the example they set, as people and as a couple, that I want to continue moving forward and helping others, in the same way they do.

I'm not sure what my future looks like. I will continue to enjoy the journey, though. What I do know is that there is so much more to it than what has happened already. Being in the NFL is one thing, and I celebrate it, but the lessons I learned there, and the person I have become since – that is what's so much more important to me.

There are so many more pages to fill, but for now, I can only move forward with that goal to share my experiences to help others deal with whatever this crazy life continues to throw at all of us. Teamwork, friendship, faith (be that in religion or in each other), and empathy can give any of us the power to overcome and find peace. I wish you luck.

Leave No One Behind.

ACKNOWLEDGMENTS

I would like to thank my family first – my mother, Rhonda, my father, Bruce, and my sisters, Laurel and Eleana – for their unwavering support through my journey.

Marshawn Lynch, Kyle Walker, Marquel Blackwell and Yusuf Shakir, thank you for reading and endorsing my book.

Thank you to Leo Moynihan for the hours spent listening to me and helping me tell my story. Thank you to Andrea Marchiano for helping me carefully edit it.

And Adam Shaw, Trigger Publishing and TriggerHub, thank you for providing me a platform to share my story, help others and move closer to my goal to Leave No One Behind.

REFERENCES

1. Associated Press. (2013, August 18). *B.J. Daniels to see more snaps*. ESPN. https://www.espn.co.uk/nfl/trainingcamp13/story/_/id/9579737/bj-daniels-climbing-san-francisco-49ers-quarterback-depth-chart
2. Abrams, J., Belson, K., & Jeter, J. (2021, April 9). *The mystery of why a foundering football player killed a family*. The New York Times. https://www.nytimes.com/2021/04/09/sports/football/phillip-adams-shooting-nfl-player.html
3. Peter, J. (2021, April 9). *Ex-NFL player Phillip Adams' "mental health degraded fast and terribly bad," says sister*. USA Today. https://eu.usatoday.com/story/sports/nfl/2021/04/08/phillip-adams-football-ex-nfl-players-mental-health-degraded-fast/7146442002/

TRIGGERHUB IS ONE OF THE MOST ELITE AND SCIENTIFICALLY PROVEN FORMS OF MENTAL HEALTH INTERVENTION

Trigger Publishing is the leading independent mental health and wellbeing publisher in the UK and US. Our collection of bibliotherapeutic books and the power of lived experience change lives forever. Our courageous authors' lived experiences and the power of their stories are scientifically endorsed by independent federal, state and privately funded research in the US. These stories are intrinsic elements in reducing stigma, making those with poor mental health feel less alone, giving them the privacy they need to heal, ensuring they are guided by the essential steps to kick-start their own journeys to recovery, and providing hope and inspiration when they need it most.

Clinical and scientific research conducted by assistant professor Dr. Kristin Kosyluk and her highly acclaimed team in the Department of Mental Health Law & Policy at the University of South Florida (USF), as well as complementary research by her peers across the US, has independently verified the power of lived experience as a core component in achieving mental health prosperity. Their findings categorically confirm lived experience as a leading method in treating those struggling with poor mental health by significantly reducing stigma and the time it takes for them to seek help, self-help or signposting if they are struggling.

Delivered through TriggerHub, our unique online portal and smartphone app, we make our library of bibliotherapeutic titles and other vital resources accessible to individuals and organizations anywhere, at any time and with complete privacy, a crucial element of recovery. As such, TriggerHub is the primary recommendation across the UK and US for the delivery of lived experiences.

At Trigger Publishing and TriggerHub, we proudly lead the way in making the unseen become seen. We are dedicated to humanizing mental health, breaking stigma and challenging outdated societal values to create real action and impact. Find out more about our world-leading work with lived experience and bibliotherapy via triggerhub.com, or by joining us on:

- 🐦 @triggerhub_
- 🇫 @triggerhub.org
- 📷 @triggerhub_

Dr. Kristin Kosyluk, Ph.D., is an assistant professor in the Department of Mental Health Law & Policy at USF, a faculty affiliate of the Louis de la Parte Florida Mental Health Institute, and director of the STigma Action Research (STAR) Lab. Find out more about Dr. Kristin Kosyluk, her team and their work by visiting:

USF Department of Mental Health Law & Policy:
www.usf.edu/cbcs/mhlp/index.aspx

USF College of Behavioral and Community Sciences:
www.usf.edu/cbcs/index.aspx

STAR Lab: www.usf.edu/cbcs/mhlp/centers/star-lab/

GET THE TRIGGERHUB APP

POWERED BY LIVED EXPERIENCE

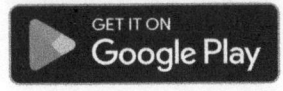

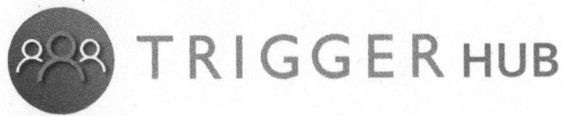

GET THE TRIGGERHUB APP

POWERED BY LIVED EXPERIENCE

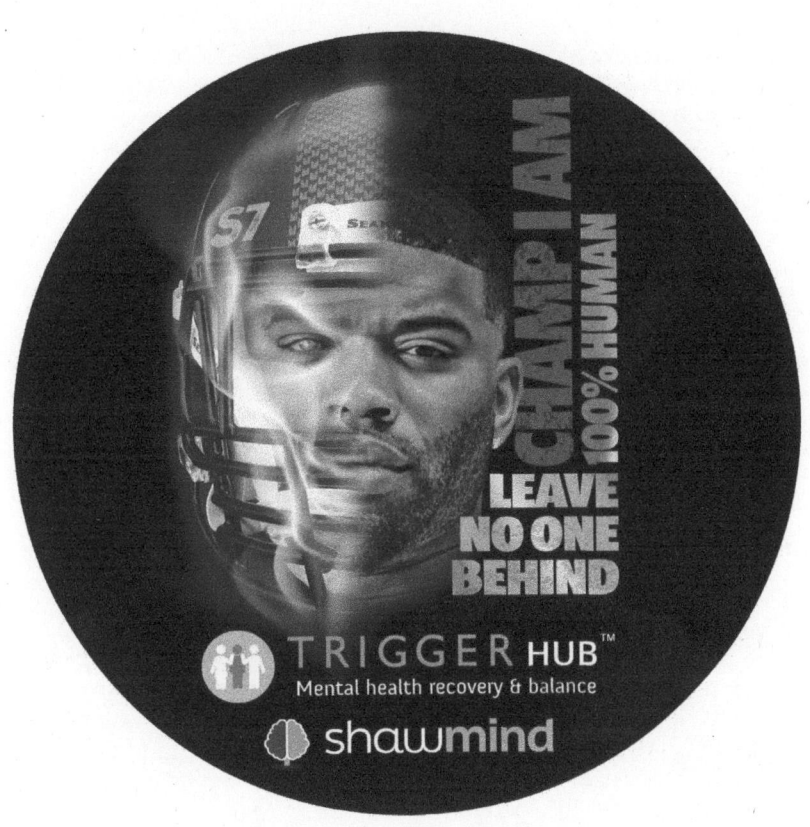

For more information, visit BJ-Super7.com